COATED WITH
FUR

A Vet's Life

D0974661

COATED WITH

FUR

A Vet's Life

KRISTEN NELSON, D.V.M.

Published by:

Veterinary Creative L.L.C.

Dedication

*This book is dedicated to all the wonderful animals and
people with whom I have worked.
May love, joy and good health fill your days.*

*I also dedicate this book to my husband, Steve.
Thanks for your neverending love, support and acceptance
of all the creatures I adopt. You are the pick of the litter!*

Contents

1. Our First Patient *1*

2. Setting up the Clinic *9*

3. Ivan's Hotspot *16*

4. Genevieve, MVC Mascot *23*

5. Allie Rescues a Cat *33*

6. Bridget Lacerates Her Paw *40*

7. Scruffy Fights for Life *46*

8. Owner's Intuition *56*

9. Nasty Animals *65*

10. Lucifer *76*

11. Cosmo Saves Us *83*

12. Blake's Christmas Puppy *90*

13. Oscar the Parrot *97*

14. Moe the Ferret *104*

15. Genevieve's Spay *114*

16. Butch the Alpha Pup *125*

17. Puppy Hit by Car *133*

18. Emily the Guinea Pig *141*

19. Sugar and Spice, Maltese Sisters *151*

20. Butch Revisited *161*

Contents.

21. Rusty the Blood Donor *166*

22. Sugar's PCV Falls *173*

23. Elvira the Snake *181*

24. Chewy the Gerbil *190*

25. Trudy, U.S. Customs Canine Officer *198*

26. Fourteen Puppies *212*

27. Cow Doc *220*

28. Emergency of the Male Variety *230*

29. Goodbye, Chewy *237*

30. Miracle of Life *247*

Acknowledgments
254

About the Author
256

Disclaimer

This book is about the wonderful animals and people I met upon opening a veterinary practice in Burnsville, Minnesota in 1992. With the exception of my own family and pets, I changed the names and other identifying characteristics to preserve confidentiality. Any similarity between details as they appear in this book and actual people or pets is strictly coincidental.

CHAPTER 1

Our First Patient

This was not how I dreamed it.

"Kris, you have two dogs hit-by-car," said my frantic husband, Steve, over the phone. "It's bad."

I felt my heart race. I was standing in the parking lot of a hardware store in Burnsville, Minnesota. The clinic wasn't open for business yet. The landlord had given me the key that very morning. Most of my supplies would not arrive until next week. Naturally, all of the nearby hospitals were closed and the emergency clinic was 20 minutes away.

"I'll be right there," I told Steve. A combination of training and experience helped me stay calm, but I had no sense what could be done under the circumstances. In an exaggerated fashion, I motioned my father, Gordon Lindstrom, to head for the car. He pushed a shopping cart full of supplies through potholes as I ran ahead and opened the trunk. We unloaded bags of brushes, paint, tape, light bulbs, pipes and garbage bags in record time and sped off.

Driving along the Minnesota River, we raced toward the clinic without a word. I typically gaze at the maple and oak trees lining the boulevard or look for waterfowl resting on the banks. But today, I kept my eyes on the road and tried to ignore the pit forming in my stomach. I considered my resources; I had fluids, catheters and a few emergency drugs on hand. Hopefully, they would be enough.

When we reached the clinic, I slammed my car to a stop next to a large pickup truck. The half-ton Chevy dwarfed my Ford Probe. Through the glass door, I saw an Australian cattle dog lying in the middle of the lobby with my family surrounding him. White foam poured from his mouth. Allie Knutson, my 24-year-old technician, knelt by the dog's head, holding an oxygen mask over his nose and mouth. The sparkling new anesthesia machine towered over her. A red first-aid kit sat on the floor by her side.

I knelt by the dog. A glassy stare covered his face. I touched the inner corner of his eye with my finger, but he didn't blink. His chest heaved up and down as he fought for air with all of his remaining strength. I reached under his hind leg to check the pulse, pressing my fingertips against the leg in search of the femoral artery. It's usually easy to find because the large vessel runs along the inner aspect of the femur. But this dog was in severe shock. Because his heart was having a hard time pumping blood through his body, his pulse was weak and rapid. We had to act fast. I feared the worst.

"Allie, let me see his gums," I ordered. She removed the mask from the dog's mouth and pulled back his lip, revealing a sick shade of blue. It should have been pink, but the color confirmed my analysis. This poor dog was starving for oxygen. An experienced technician, Allie replaced the mask and held up a catheter. "Is an 18-gauge OK?"

I nodded and took the catheter. My hands trembled as I removed the plastic guard. Through many years of school and medical practice I had placed more of these than I could recall. But today, with a new clinic, few resources and my family standing vigil – afraid for me and the dog – it was different. Allie slid her hand around the dog's elbow. She used her fingers as a tourniquet to block the flow of blood. In healthy animals, the vein distends from the backup of blood, but with this injured animal, the vein was invisible despite Allie's clip job. I pumped the paw a few times and splashed more rubbing alcohol over the prep site. I was happy to see the ever-so-faint outline of a vein appear down the center of the dog's leg between the wrist and elbow.

"His pressure is awful," I muttered. I pumped the paw again with my left hand and felt his leg with the fingertips of my right hand. "I can barely feel it."

I held the catheter over the vein with the tip hovering above the dog's leg. "Lord, help me," I prayed as it penetrated the skin. I threaded the catheter up the leg and waited. Allie and I froze in place, our eyes focused on the catheter protruding from the leg. A moment passed, then blood appeared. I slid the stylet out and capped it off.

"Nice stick, Dr. Nelson," Allie said, handing me a piece of white medical tape. I could feel my muscles release just a little. I wrapped the tape around the catheter and then securely around the dog's leg. Allie prepared a bag of Lactated Ringer's, a sterile solution used to replace fluid lost by the body. She handed the bag to my sister, Debbie Welch, with the firm instruction to hold it high to increase the flow rate. Then Allie allowed clear fluid to rush from the bag down the tubing and onto the floor. Once the air bubbles were gone, she handed the end of the drip set to me. I removed the plug from the catheter and replaced it with the fluid line.

"Now," I said in a tone accentuated by the massive amount of adrenaline coursing through me. Allie opened the valve, and fluid rushed out of the bag into the dog's leg. I turned my attention to his respiration. The dog fought for every breath, each one lifted his feet off the ground. I had to find out what was making him breathe like this. I asked Steve to find the stethoscope.

It seemed like an eternity before the stethoscope appeared. I placed the bell on the dog's chest and heard the air rushing in and out of the trachea like a wind tunnel, so loud it drowned out all the normal lung sounds.

I looked at the only stranger in the room, the dog's owner, and said, "This does not sound good." What color remained drained from the owner's face. He clung to the reception counter for support.

"I'm worried your dog has a pneumothorax," I said. "That means he has air in his chest."

I paused to collect my thoughts. My mind raced back to veterinary school and all I learned about pneumothorax. In normal animals and people, air flows down the trachea into the lungs and back out on exhalation. The system works because the space around the lungs is a vacuum. It's empty, devoid of pressure.

I turned to the owner. "I think the impact of the car damaged his lungs, and air leaked into his chest. His vacuum is gone, and he can't breathe." I pushed the oxygen mask back and lifted the dog's lip to check on his color. There was no change, despite the fluids.

"I need to tap his chest," I exclaimed as much to myself as to anyone. Turning to the owner, I said; "We need to remove the excess air. I will stick a needle into his chest and pull the air out. Is that OK?" I looked at the man for his response. He slumped over the counter with his head in his hands.

Often the hardest part of veterinary medicine is dealing with people. Giving owners time to make decisions is always hard for me, especially with critical patients like this one. This dog did not have the luxury of time. I looked at Steve and wrung my hands. Debbie and Allie exchanged a concerned glance. What was he waiting for?

Finally, the man straightened and faced me. His eyes glistened with tears under the clinic lights. "Do what you think is best, Doc," he whispered and looked down at his leather cowboy boots. "I don't want to lose Cody." He raised his hand to forehead, closed his eyes and made the Sign of the Cross over his chest. When he finished, he kissed his fingers and touched the dog's back.

Allie sprang into action. She clipped a nine-by-nine-inch square patch over the dog's rib cage. Loose brown hair fell onto the floor. She disinfected the area with Betadine scrub and rinsed it with rubbing alcohol. While I donned a pair of surgical gloves, Steve grabbed a 35-milliliter syringe and a butterfly catheter from the first-aid kit. He opened the packages carefully and slid them into my gloved hands. I connected the syringe to the rubber tubing of the catheter.

As Allie finished the sterile prep, the pit returned to my stomach. If the tear in Cody's lung was large, this chest tap would not work. He'd need a chest tube with continuous suction. My suction equipment would not arrive for a week.

Allie rubbed her hands on her pants to dry off the slimy scrub. "Ready," she said. I passed the syringe to her and took a deep breath. I dreaded the feeling of the needle passing through the muscles of the chest. The professors said I would get over it with time, but in four years of practice I had not. I always thought how much it must hurt. Cody could not afford to wait for me to numb the area with lidocaine. His gums looked gray.

I felt his fifth and sixth rib with my left hand and identified the muscular space between. Grasping the special catheter by its plastic wings, I plunged the needle deep into Cody's side. The dog did not flinch. His chest continued to heave up and down with each breath.

Allie drew back the plunger on the syringe, filling it with air. When it was full, I kinked off the tubing with my left hand while holding the needle in place with my right. She disconnected the syringe and flushed the air from the chamber. "One," she counted out loud. When it was reconnected, I unfolded the tubing, and Allie pulled more air out of Cody's chest. He did not fight the chest tap at all. We repeated this over and over again. "Two, three, four." The air just kept coming. "Five, six, seven." The dog's chest continued to rise and fall. He still fought for each breath.

Worry and doubt crept into my mind. I quickly calculated how much air we had removed. Seven times 35 is about 250 milliliters, which isn't that much for an Australian cattle dog. As the amount of excess air decreased, Allie would need to pull harder on the syringe. Hopefully, she would feel resistance soon.

"Are you getting any resistance at all?" I asked desperately. She frowned.

"Eight, nine, 10." She smiled when the syringe finally became harder to pull. It dug into her fingers, leaving red marks. She rubbed them against her leg to remove the numbness and pulled again. The plunger slid halfway back and stopped. I removed the needle and reinserted it higher on Cody's chest. "Here goes 11," she said. Halfway through the next syringe, I felt a scratching sensation on the tip of the needle. Even though lung tissue is soft and elastic, it feels as rough and abrasive as steel wool during a chest tap.

"Stop," I ordered. Allie took her fingers off the plunger. I repositioned the needle and asked her to pull again. Five milliliters of air flowed into the syringe before I felt lung again. I withdrew the needle completely.

For the first time, Cody closed his mouth and inhaled through his nose. I sat back on my heels with a sigh of relief and watched his chest. His ribs moved slowly up and down with each breath, and his respiratory rate slowed to normal. Allie removed the oxygen mask from his face and pulled back his lip. A healthy pink color replaced the deathly gray tone. Cody stuck out his tongue and licked his lips.

"Whew!" I exclaimed with delight.

The man slumped over the counter again, this time washed in relief. Tears of joy streamed down his face. He pulled a red handkerchief from his pocket and wiped his eyes. Smiles spread across my family's faces. Cody could breathe again.

I removed my gloves to tend to the second dog, but didn't see it anywhere. "Weren't there two dogs?" I asked. I looked around the room, but no one answered. I distinctly remembered Steve saying there were two dogs.

Finally, Allie pointed at the truck and whispered, "Cody's buddy didn't make it. He was DOA." The somber words immediately squashed the joy I felt from seeing Cody improve. I slowly rose to my feet and stood by the man's side.

"I'm sorry about your other dog Mr. uh, Mr. ... I'm sorry, I don't even know your name." He turned to face me with his right hand extended.

"Tommy, Tommy Munson," he replied as we shook hands. "I thought they was locked-up when I left." He cleared his throat and swallowed hard. "They never seen the car. Poor Jeb." He bit his lip and sniffed loudly. Through the lobby window, I saw Jeb's body lying in the bed of the pickup. The wind ruffled his beautiful fur coat. "Cody will be heartbroken without him." He slid his thumbs into the pockets of his tightly fitting jeans.

At the sound of his name, Cody lifted his head off the floor. I returned to his side and checked his pulse. It felt strong and regular. I placed my stethoscope over his heart. Lub, dub, lub, dub echoed in my ears, its beats crisp and regular. No signs of a murmur. I moved the bell of the stethoscope around his chest. Soft sounds of air moving through his lungs replaced the harsh rattle from before.

"What happens now?" Tommy asked.

Because this was our first day and the clinic was not operational, I explained that Cody should go to the emergency clinic for continued care. He needed X-rays to check for fractured bones and bruised lungs. My machine was not set up yet. I gave Cody an injection of Demoral to control his pain and ran my fingers over his body once it took effect. I manipulated his head and front legs and, palpated the abdomen and back, searching for signs of injury. So far, so good.

When I reached his back left leg, Cody swung his head toward me, teeth exposed.

"Sorry, boy." I released the leg. Orthopedic injuries are so painful.

Allie took a muzzle out of the first-aid kit and slid it over Cody's nose. I continued to palpate his leg. The hip was swollen, probably fractured. Now it was time to examine the other side. Allie held Cody's head, Debbie had his middle, and I took the back end. On the count of three, we rolled him onto his left side on top of a thick wool blanket, the kind we all have in Minnesota. Cody yelped so loudly we all jumped.

After I examined his right side, Allie prepped his chest for a second tap. This time Cody jumped when the needle penetrated his chest. Only a few milliliters of air flowed into the syringe. Thank heavens, he would not need a chest tube. We rolled him back to his right side to take pressure off his injured left hip. Allie left him muzzled.

As I stood and stretched my back, Tommy asked, "What's the verdict, Doc?"

"I've stabilized him as best I can. Now you need to get him to the emergency clinic. I'm worried his chest might fill with air again, or he might revert into shock.

Tommy pressed his lips together and nodded. "He's a tough dog, he'll make it."

We used the blanket as a sling to carry Cody to the cab of Tommy's truck. Once he was more or less comfortable, I removed the muzzle and rubbed his nose. "Good luck Cody." He licked my hand and began to pant – it was a good sign.

Tommy promised to call with an update. As he pulled away, everyone went inside except Steve and me. We stood together silently watching him depart. Steve put his arm around my shoulder. A thousand thoughts raced through my mind. Here I was, a young veterinarian who now owned her own clinic. There was so much to do. Quite unexpectedly, we had treated our first patient. While it seemed he would make it, I was not at all certain about my clinic.

CHAPTER 2

Setting up the Clinic

E arlier that first day at 8 a.m. sharp, I pulled into the clinic parking lot in the black Ford Probe. Cleaning and paint supplies filled the car to the ceiling. My dad followed me in his pickup truck full of tools. My heart raced as I backed into a space in front of the building. We had a lot to accomplish in a short period of time.

For much of the prior year, I had spent free time searching for a clinic – a clinic of my own. I looked at several existing hospitals, but the price tag was always too high. Most owners wanted a young veterinarian who would buy into the practice a little at a time until the owner was ready to retire – the traditional method of sale. I would provide most of the labor while the older veterinarian received most of the profits.

Instead of pursuing that route, I decided to start a clinic from scratch. I had already served as medical director of a start-up. I routinely put in 10-hour days to make the clinic a success. Now, with Steve's support and encouragement, I was ready to try it on my own. I used funds we'd saved for a house down payment as seed money. Everything we owned was on the line – our cars, our furniture and our cash. Although Steve was a portfolio manager in a trust department, he was early in his career. Our future depended on my success.

After months of searching and after several potential locations fell through, I finally found a place to rent. Located in an industrial complex, the building was not much to look at from the outside. Gray cement blocks formed the exterior. Skinny floor-to-ceiling windows and glass doors interrupted the otherwise drab exterior. It was a low-slung, non-descript strip mall, the kind easily overlooked while driving down the road. In spite of the ordinary appearance, its location next to a boarding kennel was terrific. I hoped to garner business vaccinating pets for owners frantic to get out of town. Without current vaccinations for their pets, they could not board the animals.

Built in the 1970s, the original occupant transformed the raw shell into a small animal clinic with four exam rooms, a lobby and pharmacy/laboratory area in the front. The back half housed the treatment room, kennels, radiology suite and operating room. Orange paint and wild wallpaper covered the walls. The colors made a bold statement next to the dark wood cabinets and brown linoleum floors. It was groovy, I guess.

When the clinic owner moved to a new location, the facility became an emergency clinic owned by a group of local veterinarians. They kept the clinic well stocked with drugs and necessary equipment, but spent no money updating the décor. Overcome by the sight, clients used to freeze in the lobby. Now, I had one weekend to bring the space into the '90s.

"Dad, did you ever think this day would come?"

"No," he replied. He tucked the back of his plaid shirt into his dark green work pants. "I was hoping Steve would get stuck with this job. You know how I love to paint."

I offered a short prayer, then slid the key into the lock and opened the door. Tears welled up in my eyes. Unfortunately, they were not tears of joy. The room reeked. The rotten odor made my eyes water and my nose run. I covered my nose and mouth with a hand. Dad pulled a white hanky from his pocket and covered his nose.

We walked through the waiting room, into the pharmacy area. Panels from the overhead lights hung from the ceiling. The bulbs were gone, stripped from their sockets. Boxes and bags littered the room. Cabinet doors hung half-open, exposing empty shelves.

The foul odor seemed to come from the kennel. We continued through the treatment room to the doorway to the darkened kennels. I swallowed hard to fight the increasing waves of nausea. I fumbled for the light switch. Bam! A sharp crashing sound radiated through the room. The tip of my tennis shoes hit something metal lying on the floor.

Light flowed from one naked bulb that dangled over the kennels. Copper pipes littered the floor along with pieces of drywall and ceiling tiles. The prior tenant had ripped out the oxygen system. We stood frozen for a minute. Our eyes darted around the room from floor to ceiling. It looked like a war zone with debris scattered all around.

We decided to split up. Dad headed off to the radiology suite. I poked my head into the dark room used to develop X-rays. Exposed pipes with ends smashed stuck out from the walls. Glass shards lay on the floor from the safe light.

Around the corner, I spied the bathtub. A mixture of black and rusted material ran down the sides and spilled over the front edge. I stepped back to avoid a puddle. As my foot hit the floor, it slipped almost sending me to the ground. I grabbed the bathtub with both hands and regained my balance. My hands just missed the brown goo.

I turned around to see what caused my slip. More brown goo covered the floor where the freezer used to rest. The material seemed to move. My stomach jumped to my throat. I found the source of the stench: maggots!

Dad walked into the room with a flashlight in his hand. He

aimed the beam on the floor. The maggots squirmed away from the light. He clicked off the beam. "How in the world did they get here?" he asked. I shook my head, as bewildered as he was.

This was the area where the emergency clinic housed a freezer. The former veterinarians placed euthanized pets here until a service picked them up for cremation. Perhaps the freezer leaked blood onto the floor. I shivered in disgust.

"I'll take care of it as soon as I finish taking some pictures," I announced. "No one will believe me otherwise."

A former Seabee in World War II, my dad is nothing if not resourceful. Dad fashioned a small piece of wood into a doorstop and propped open the front door. Scavenging some wire from the floor to open the back door, he strung a long piece from the door handle to the railing outside. We turned the fans on high. I sprayed a mixture of bleach and water over the maggots and bathtub area. While that soaked, I cleaned the bathroom, which looked worse than a state fair Port-O-Potty. By the time Allie arrived, the maggots were a bad memory.

I met Allie through our work. Like all great veterinary technicians, she was able to run a heartworm test, set up a fecal test, fill a prescription and answer the phone all at the same time. She was game to help in any way she could, even if she was unfamiliar with what was asked or expected. I'll never forget the first time I asked her to hold an iguana. Her eyes widened at the request, but she bravely extended her hand toward the iguana's head. Thank goodness, he just lay there and let her pick him up.

Allie attacked the laboratory/pharmacy area with a vengeance. This was her domain, and she wanted it clean and well organized. With her curly brown hair pulled back into a ponytail, she was all business as she threw out the yellowed shelf liners and scrubbed the bottom of the shelves and drawers.

When Steve's parents, Dr. Bob and Barb Nelson, arrived, Barb teamed up with Allie to clean. My father-in-law, an industrial veterinarian, took a day off from work to help. In preparation for painting, he taped the walls in the front exam room that I decided to convert into a children's play area. I hauled loads of garbage to the dumpster. In between loads, I made a list for what became an endless series of runs to the hardware store. Fluorescent light bulbs and garbage bags topped it.

Suddenly, a loud crash followed by the sound of breaking glass came from the back of the building. Allie jumped and almost fell off the stepladder. Bob poked his head out of the kids' room with a concerned look on his face.

"What was that?" he asked.

"I think Dad dropped a light bulb." I rubbed my forehead with my hand. "Maybe I should get two boxes of light bulbs." Everyone laughed. I walked to the back with a broom and dustpan.

Upon my return, the lobby buzzed with activity. Blue tape was everywhere, along the doorways, around windows and covering electrical outlets. A stepladder stood in the middle of the lobby with the shelf extended. Debbie sat on the ground next to an opened can of snow-white paint.

My sister and I were not very close growing up. With nine years between us, she was a teenager when I was in grade school. I was likely more of an annoyance than a sister. She married and moved out of our parents' house after her first year of college. I carried vague memories of her from those years ... watching her get ready for prom, eating Grandmother's Swedish pancakes with her and fighting over the couch in the den. She always won because of her long fingernails. As adults, we grew closer, and it brought me joy to have her there this day.

"The paint is ready." Debbie poured a moderate amount into the two paint trays sitting next to the can. Dad plunged a fluffy pink roller in one tray and placed the tray on the stepladder. He then picked up the ladder, made one step toward the small exam room and put it down.

"What's wrong, Dad?" Debbie asked.

"I forgot to get a rag." As he turned away from the ladder, his shoulder caught the corner of the paint tray.

"Dad, the ..." Debbie yelled. The paint tray tumbled down the ladder's side, landing with a crash. A wave of white paint sprayed over the counter, down the front and onto the floor. The paint tray landed face down on the floor just off the drop cloth.

Debbie and I grabbed a roll of paper towels from the counter and frantically tried to mop up the mess. Dad stood in shock. White speckles covered his work pants and threatened to drip onto his leather work shoes. Allie ran behind the counter for more paper towels. She threw two rolls over the counter into my hands before disappearing into the back.

"I'm sorry, Krissy."

"No worries, Dad. Debbie and I will have this cleaned up in no time."

I scooped up the excess paint with my hands and poured it back into the paint tray. Allie gave Dad a towel and told him to clean up before the paint dried. Once he was gone, Debbie and I began to giggle. In the coming days, we often would look at each other and giggle even more.

"I could have predicted this would happen," she smirked.

I sat back on my heels and squeezed the rag into the bucket. "As soon as we get this cleaned up, I'm going to make a run to the hardware store." Allie pulled a small notepad and pen from her back pocket. She jotted down a few items on the first page, ripped it out and handed it to me.

"Is she always that prepared?" Debbie asked.

I nodded. "That's why I hired her. She's really good." Allie beamed.

After the paint incident, I made a management decision and re-assigned Dad to plumbing. I like to think of my dad as a modern-day renaissance man. He was a carpenter and roofing contractor first and foremost but also knew the basics of plumbing, welding, masonry and electrical work. Now his skills would be tested at my new clinic.

When I formulated my business plan, most of the money went

to equipment, supplies and pharmaceuticals. I allotted a small sum for painting and repair. Since it was a functioning clinic before my rental, I thought most of the work would be cosmetic and rather inexpensive. Instead, we encountered a badly damaged space that required time and money to repair. Both were in short supply.

CHAPTER 3

Ivan's Hotspot

As I arrived at the clinic, sounds of football practice echoed in the distance. Cheers punctuated with shrill whistles pierced the morning air. I stood next to my car and watched groups of young men dressed in dirty white practice uniforms run up and down the field. Farther up the hill, the brick buildings of Burnsville High School gleamed in the morning light.

The wall clock read 7:45 when I flipped on the lights in the lobby. The clinic had changed dramatically since that first day. Crisp white walls with blue accents replaced the orange and brown décor of a decade gone by. Wooden chairs with thick blue cushions lined the block walls. Two framed posters of dog and cat breeds hung above the chairs, providing visual interest. These charts were a favorite of my clients who enjoyed finding their pets' lineage among the illustrations.

A large potted plant, a Norfolk pine that had once been a Christmas tree for Steve and me, sat in front of the waiting room window. When we first moved back to Minnesota from Ohio, we lived in an apartment on the north side of the Twin Cities. The apartment complex outlawed real Christmas trees to prevent fires, so Steve and I hung ornaments and a garland on the potted plant. It reminded me of Charlie Brown's Christmas tree.

I placed my coat and bag in the office closet and checked the answering machine. Unfortunately, there were no messages; business was slow. I set a goal of seeing at least one client a day. Yesterday, the big transaction was a bag of cat food. I still counted it toward the goal.

Walking through the kennel doorway, a dull thud from the front of the building stopped me in my tracks. I hurried up front and saw a man walking across the parking lot with a Doberman by his side. The dog's silver choke collar sparkled like a fine piece of jewelry.

"Excuse me," I called out. The man stopped, and the dog instantly sat by his feet on his left. "May I help you?" He turned and walked back toward the building. Again, the dog heeled in perfect unison.

"I thought this was an emergency clinic," he responded.

"They moved out last month. But I'd be happy to help you." I smiled and introduced myself, trying to mask my desperation. The man looked familiar. He wore a leather jacket and tweed pants that showed off his athletic body. His kind eyes seemed to twinkle when he smiled, reminding me of Santa Claus.

Introducing himself as Rich Harris, he showed me a circular area of moist, pink skin without any hair on Ivan's rear end. Rich explained that Ivan suffered from hotspots, a staph infection of the skin. He had licked the last one into a bloody mess. The poor dog had to wear an Elizabethan or e-collar for weeks while it healed. Like most animals, he hated the big lampshade on his head. He ran into the door-jambs and chipped off the paint. Rich pulled up his sleeve and looked at the gold Rolex strapped to his wrist. He wanted the dog treated before the infection got worse, but he had to be at work by 9.

I explained that my technician would not arrive for another hour. If he wouldn't mind helping me, I'd be happy to look at his dog. He agreed and walked into the lobby with Ivan heeling in perfect position. Ivan's eyes darted anxiously around the room as Rich filled-out the new-client questionnaire. Ivan placed his head on the counter and whined. He knew a veterinary clinic from a mile away and wanted no part of it.

I escorted them into the large pharmacy/laboratory area. The extra space in the main room, gave me plenty of room to work on the big dog. Ivan stood like a statue for the physical examination. I started at his head and worked my way to his tail. Thank goodness, I did not find additional hotspots.

"OK, Buddy, you need to lie down," I instructed the dog. Ivan continued to look at his owner without moving. Rich laughed and commanded him to lie down in German. On the word "platz" he reluctantly lay down with the hotspot buried beneath his body.

"He's such a brat sometimes," Rich joked. Together, we rolled him over. A low rumble emanated from Ivan's throat. I was glad I had his rear end. Rich shook his head and told him to knock it off. Ivan lifted his lip, looked at his owner and then let it drop into place again.

With Ivan on the proper side, I clipped off all the hair around the hotspot. When I tried to clip the hair right on the margin of the hotspot, the large dog raised his head and growled again. Rich quickly pulled Ivan's head back into his lap. The faint smell of men's cologne filled the room. Ivan wiggled his nose and sneezed. This part always hurts. Slime from the moist infection gums the hair down to the skin. I sprayed some lube on the clipper and continued. The gooey hair piled up on the top of the metal blade as I worked.

"You and Ivan seem so familiar," I replied once the clip job was complete. I picked up a piece of gauze soaked in iodine disinfectant. "Have we met before?" Rich nodded and smiled.

"You replaced his I.V. catheter several months ago," he replied.

Now I remembered this dog. Rich and his wife, Linda, brought Ivan in for a new catheter. Ivan suffered from severe vomiting and bloody diarrhea and couldn't keep anything down, even water. His regular vet placed a catheter and treated him with I.V. fluids during the day. At night, Linda administered his fluids. After two days, Ivan ripped-out the catheter when Rich left him unattended to answer the phone. Rich returned to find saline dripped on the carpeting. Blood oozed from Ivan's leg where the catheter had been. I was the unlucky veterinarian who got to reset it.

Schutzhund-trained dogs always make me nervous. Schutzhund for dogs is like martial arts for people. These dogs learn how to defend themselves and their people. The German program starts with obedience and then progresses to protection work. After the basics – sit and down, or "sitz" and "platz," – the dogs learn bite and attack skills. The bad guy wears a steel arm protector marked with a target over the forearm. Over time, the dog learns to clamp on to the "target" and hold until directed to release by the handler. At the end of the program, many graduates go on to a career in crime prevention.

Rich had held Ivan for me, while I placed a new catheter. I remembered working on his front leg, while his enormous teeth hovered inches above my hand. The dog had growled at me then, too. Linda had assured me he was only talking and that he would not bite unless commanded. I did not share her certainty. The dog's intense stare had made me feel like a sitting duck.

"Oh, now I remember," I said. I stopped scrubbing the hotspot and rinsed the area with water. Ivan looked at me with his big brown eyes. The cool water brought relief from the itchy infection. I blotted the area dry and sprayed a topical anesthetic over the inflamed skin. Ivan flinched in response. The medicine burned at first but numbed the area in a few seconds. He smelled like a medicine chest. It overpowered his owner's cologne.

Ivan licked his lips, exposing his large canine teeth. He swung his head toward the hotspot with his tongue sticking out of his mouth. Rich grabbed his snout and pushed it to the side. I jerked my hand out of the way. Ivan licked the air, narrowly missing his intended target. His neck muscles bulged beneath his slick black coat as he tried again. I distracted him with an ear rub until the medicine took effect. He moaned with delight and closed his eyes.

While I prepared the dog's discharge medicine, Rich let Ivan off lead to explore. He ignored the medicine cabinets, but enjoyed sniffing the racks of prescription food. Our clinic birds fascinated him. He stood in front of their cages with his eyes darting from one cage to another. The first cage held Bongo, a bright green Amazon parrot with a yellow head, who suffered from horrible eyesight. She stayed high on her perch away from Ivan's eager nose.

Oscar, a medium-sized macaw in the middle cage ignored the eager canine as well. The bird turned his back to the annoying dog, but his long tail feathers stuck through the bars under the food cup. Ivan eagerly sniffed the feathers until Oscar squawked loudly. Ivan jumped back with a look of surprise.

Windsor, the little cockatiel in the last cage, did the opposite. Windsor slid down the bars of his cage and perched on a feed cup, eye-to-eye with Ivan. Windsor might have been the smallest bird in my collection, but he had the biggest heart. No Doberman was going to intimidate him. The gray bird with orange circles on his cheeks spread his wings out to the side and fanned the yellow crest of feathers on the top of his head in defiance. He dared Ivan to put his nose within reach of his sharp little beak. Ivan stared back as if to say, "Are you kidding me?"

"Careful, Ivan," I called to him. "Windsor can really bite. I know from experience."

Rich walked over to Ivan, clipped a leash to his collar and pulled him away. Windsor strutted back and forth at the bottom of his cage with his crest held high. A low chortle rattled from his throat. He showed Ivan who was boss.

I handed a medicine bottle labeled Minnesota Veterinary Center to Rich. Ivan thought it might be a toy and tried to grab it. Rich responded with a laugh. Obviously, the over-sized Doberman could do no wrong in his eyes. When I unscrewed the top of the cookie jar an overwhelming beef smell escaped. Ivan was next to me in a split second. He licked his lips and nosed my elbow in encouragement.

After the OK command from Rich, Ivan gently removed the cookie from the palm of my hand. His lips felt like velvet. Two chomps later, the cookie was a distant memory. Ivan barked and begged for more, staring at the cookie jar. I petted his head instead, not wanting to upset his delicate stomach with too many treats.

While I wrote in Ivan's medical record, he rubbed against my leg. Then he turned around and backed into my leg. I felt his rear end slide down until his butt rested on my shoe. His hip bone crushed my foot into the floor. A numbing sensation spread through my toes, which tingled as if they were frozen. I tried to pull my foot out, but Ivan just pushed with more force.

"Ah, Ivan," I stammered. "What's with sitting on my foot?"

Rich started to giggle. "It means he likes you," he said. I gave him a quizzical glance. I had never experienced this with any other dog. My foot ached. "Really," he continued. Ivan's eyes pleaded with me to believe him. "He only sits on your foot if he likes you."

"Well, I like you, too." I patted Ivan's head. I couldn't feel my toes anymore. "But I would like you better if you weren't sitting on my foot." I pushed his rear off my foot with both hands. Ivan gazed at me with angelic eyes as he tried to sit on my other foot. I pulled it out of the way just in time. His rear landed on the floor with a thud. He looked at me again and wagged his stump of a tail. Ivan was a charmer. Rich called him over to his side. Ivan took one last look before obeying. I couldn't tell if he was looking at me or the cookie jar.

As I escorted Rich and Ivan back to the lobby, Ivan pranced along, seeming to float above the floor. Before opening the door, I proudly gave Rich a business card. He tucked it into his wallet with a promise to call if the hotspot was not gone in three days. Ivan stared out the front door, leaving nose-prints all over the glass.

Rich thanked me for the help, happy that he had enough time to drop Ivan off at home before heading to work. When I reminded him to put the e-collar on the dog as soon as possible, he promised that Ivan would be wearing it before they left the parking lot.

"And congratulations on the clinic," Rich added. "It must be very exciting to open a business of your own."

I smiled and nodded. As an employee, the thought of owning my own business and running the show seemed glamorous. Now I was starting to worry about paying the bills and meeting the biweekly payroll. Freedom, it seems, has its costs.

Still, it was a good start to the day. At least I had one transaction out of the way early.

CHAPTER 4

Genevieve, MVC Mascot

Allie roared into the parking lot in her fire-engine-red sports car. Large black fuzzy dice with red dots hung from the rearview mirror. She pulled her hair back into a ponytail before entering the building. High school boys walking down the sidewalk stopped to gaze as she strode across the parking lot in her hot pink scrubs. At precisely 9 a.m., she entered the lobby.

"Good morning, Allie. You seem to have a fan club," I observed. The group of awkward teenagers still stood on the sidewalk, staring at our building.

"Please." She stretched the word into four syllables. "I like mature men." She rolled her eyes and tossed back her head. A dark blue sedan pulled-up in front of the clinic. Allie threw her bag under the counter and prepared to greet our first appointment of the morning, Winston. We weren't really sure why the curly Airedale was here. When Harold Warren had called, he mumbled something about bobsledding.

Allie escorted Winston and his owner into the dog room. Sky-blue paint covered the bottom half of the walls with bright white on top. A wide wallpaper border bridged the gap. On the border,

Yellow Labrador puppies played with duck decoys and hunting whistles. An oak peninsula cabinet that served as both exam table and storage unit jutted into the middle of the room. The blue laminate top matched the blue paint.

I entered the room from the back door. The handsome dog sat on the table with Harold standing behind him. Winston looked like a poster puppy for Airedale Terriers with his rusty brown coat. Black hair covered his back, the shape resembling a saddle. He sat with his head up and feet perfectly aligned in front of him. As sometimes happens with owners and pets, Harold Warren bore a striking resemblance to Winston. Tight curls of black hair fell across his forehead. He stood straight with shoulders back as if a book balanced on his head.

"Good morning," I greeted the pair. Harold nodded. "What can we do for you today?" Although Allie had inquired several times in different ways, the reason for Winston's visit remained a mystery. Harold mentioned bobsledding and then clammed up. He looked so uncomfortable that Allie quit pressing. Now it was up to me to solve the puzzle.

Harold looked down at his dog. He shifted back and forth on his feet. "Winston is bobsledding again," he whispered. There was that word again. I asked various questions designed to discern his cryptic meaning. Harold answered them all politely but continued to describe the problem as bobsledding. After four minutes of this, the owner was ready to get on with it. I got the impression that he was beginning to wonder about my abilities as a veterinarian.

I examined Winston from top to bottom without any clues. The pressure mounted as I tried in vain to find anything that would help me overcome our communication barrier.

With the examination over, Harold looked at me expectantly. I looked at him one more time. Winston studied my face earnestly. He seemed to be waiting on me, too. I inhaled deeply and tried to collect my thoughts.

Before I could speak, Winston sprang into action. He used his front legs to drag his rear end on the table and, like magic, the diagnosis was clear. The dog needed his anal glands emptied. In four years as a veterinarian, I have heard people describe this condition in many ways ... scooting, dragging, skidding but never bobsledding. This was a first. I guess I should have known, this being Minnesota, king of winter sports. Two quick squeezes later, Winston was clean as a whistle. His bobsledding days were over until his anal glands filled up again.

The condition is painful. Dogs and cats both have the sacs, which are similar to the glands on a skunk. In veterinary college a professor told us there was "a lot of money in anal sacs." Now I was a beneficiary of this truism. Winston was visibly relieved, and Harold was happy.

The next appointment was a cat with an ear problem. A couple of months ago, Bob Williams noticed his cat scratching one ear. Spaatz sat on the table, his right ear folded back against his head. Scabs surrounded the hairless base of his ear. His constant scratching resulted in skin that resembled hamburger. Inside, swollen pink tissue bulged into the ear canal, and clumps of dark brown material covered the ear's mucosa. Spaatz's black coat looked unkempt, with matted clumps of hair here and there. His white feet and chin looked dull under the fluorescent lights of the exam room.

According to his owner, the ear problem transformed Spaatz from a loving companion to a grumpy Gus. He stopped interacting with his family. Instead of greeting Bob at the door when he returned from work, Spaatz hid under the bed. He did not want attention. The night before, he picked at his dinner and refused this morning's breakfast. His now desperate owner was at his wits' end.

Spaatz growled when I touched his ear. He knew from experience what came next, and he wanted no part of it. Allie wrapped him in a large blanket. With only his head showing, he looked like a "kitty burrito."

I placed the smallest cone I had on the otoscope and carefully inserted it into the affected ear. Allie held him down with both hands. Slowly, I advanced it through the vertical part of the ear canal to the horizontal part. White dots scurried across my field of view. A microscopic examination of some of the brown debris confirmed my suspicion. Poor Spaatz had ear mites. The swab was loaded with them! I felt my scalp itch in sympathy for the kitty. That always happens when I think about mites, ticks, fleas, lice or maggots.

I cleaned his ear as best I could and instilled three drops of an antiparasitic medicine. The owner scheduled a recheck in two weeks.

As soon as Spaatz left the building, Allie stormed into my office. Doors slammed in her wake. Her green eyes flashed with anger. I hoped I had not done something wrong. Allie had spent several days developing a good system for the front office. Did I mess up her system this morning with Ivan?

"Remember the family who brought in two cats for health certificates?" I nodded. "The woman just called and said they need to get rid of their lovebird because they are moving to South Carolina." She placed her hands on her hips. "How can people do that?" She barreled on before I could answer. "Get rid of a pet just because they are moving. You just buy a carrier and take your pets with you." She waved her arms in the air as she spoke. "How could they bring the cats, yet leave a little bird behind?"

I sat back in my chair and watched Allie pace back and forth. Frustration spewed as she discussed the nature of irresponsible owners and her view of them.

When she finished, I concurred. I have seen people surrender animals for a variety of reasons – stupid reasons in my opinion – at the local shelter. One couple got rid of a Great Dane puppy because it grew over the 25 pound weight limit at their apartment building. I wanted to ask them if they had ever seen a Great Dane before they bought one? Members of this breed usually weigh more than 100 pounds at maturity. What were they thinking?

Another person abandoned a Persian cat because it shed too much. I shook my head as I thought of the suffering this causes the animals. They suffer because their people are irresponsible. It makes me want to scream.

"So what's going to happen to the bird?" I asked.

"I don't know." Her anger continued to boil. She clenched her fists until her knuckles turned white. "The lady said they might let the bird go. She's too busy packing to find a home for him."

That's a death sentence in this climate. The poor little bird would freeze to death. I looked at my own birds playing in their cages. Over the years, I had amassed a collection of misfits no one wanted. Each had its own personality, likes and dislikes that made it special. Why not add one more?

"Allie, call the lady and tell her to bring the bird here." I smiled at Allie. "He can hang out with the others until we find him a home." She nodded but did not return the smile. Allie considered her pets an integral part of the family. She felt there should be a law preventing these irresponsible people from adopting more animals. I agreed.

"Hello," a deep voice called from the lobby. "Is anyone home?"

A minute later, Dad poked his head into the office. He wore his customary outfit, work pants and a plaid shirt. He usually carried a toolbox with him, but today he had a small blue carrier.

"Look who I brought with me," he said, holding the carrier in front of his chest. A young tortoiseshell kitten huddled at the front of the carrier. The stripes on her forehead formed a perfect 'M'. Her yellow-green eyes took in everything around her.

"Genny!" I got up and took the carrier from my dad.

Two months before, I was filling in for a friend on the north side of town. A man entered the clinic with a cardboard box in his hands. Inside, a newborn kitten lay motionless, missing its back right leg. Everything below the hock was gone. The man said he found the kitten behind a dumpster with the leg missing and wanted it put out of its misery. The receptionist took the box to the back and asked me what I wanted to do.

When I opened the box, the kitten lifted her head and opened her mouth. No sound came out. She tried again with the same result. The kitten's fur coat had stripes of orange, brown and black with a touch of white. Her eyes were sealed shut. I felt awful watching the kitten's silent cries for help.

I cupped the infant in my hands. She felt cold and limp. Moist, pink remnants of the umbilical cord still clung to her navel. The kitten was an hour old at most. I turned her over, hoping the man had exaggerated the extent of her injuries. Unfortunately, he had not. The kitten's entire foot was gone, severed at the hock. What was left of the leg was a bloody mess. The sight of it made even me, a veterinarian seasoned in trauma, a little queasy. The kitten had lost a lot of blood.

When I questioned the man, he told me a different story. He said his cat gave birth to a litter of kittens. The others were all normal, but this one was a freak. The man wanted it put out of its misery. Looking at the injury and listening to the owner, I drew a mental picture of what probably had occurred. At the kitten's birth, a piece of placenta wrapped around the back leg. The mother cat tried to lick it off. When that failed, she chewed it off along with the kitten's foot. Although this happens sometimes, I shuddered at the thought.

When I explained what I thought really happened, the man felt insulted. His cat would never do anything like that. I explained that it was instinct, not a character flaw that motivated her. He refused to believe me and also declined to take the kitten back to its mother. I felt the kitten lift her head. She nuzzled my hand once and collapsed. Her skinny abdomen told me she had not nursed since birth.

"Could I keep her?" I blurted out. The man looked at me with an icy stare. An evil grin spread across his face. I worried he would say no just to get back at me for suggesting his cat damaged the kitten's leg. He started to say no when I interrupted him. "It would save you the euthanasia fee."

He looked at me and said, "suit yourself." He rattled the keys in his pocket and left without giving the kitten another glance.

I rushed to treat the newborn. Even with great care, the odds were stacked against her. I threaded a tube down her throat and into her stomach. As newborns do, she purred when warm milk flowed down the tube. Next, I rubbed her rear end with a warm, moist cotton ball. Newborn puppies and kittens cannot void without prompting. Three cotton balls later, I finished the job.

With the basics out of the way, I turned my attention to her leg. I cleaned the exposed muscles and tendons, then covered them with lube to keep them moist. I wrapped the stump in bandages for protection. After an injection of antibiotics, the kitten slept peacefully in her box, surrounded by improvised hot water bottles – exam gloves filled with hot water and knotted off at the wrist. In a pinch, these work fine.

For the next two weeks, Steve and I fed the baby orphan every two hours, 'round the clock. Since she was still too weak to nurse from a bottle, Steve held her while I passed a feeding tube down her throat. Her tummy swelled from the kitten milk replacer. She purred happily until we moved on to the next step. She did not like the warm cotton ball treatment and voiced her displeasure in precious squeaks.

"How could such a beautiful baby produce such nasty stuff?" Steve wondered. It was a feeling shared by parents worldwide.

To compensate for her small size, we felt the kitten needed a big name. For a few days we bantered about possibilities. Nothing seemed to suit the little princess until Steve thought of the name Genevieve. It stuck.

After five weeks of round-the-clock feedings, I was exhausted. Genny, refused to eat on her own even though she possessed sharp baby teeth. I offered all kinds of food, both canned and dry, but she refused. A syringe full of warm kitten milk was what she wanted. She placed her lips on the end of the syringe and sucked with all her might. She could drain a three-cc syringe in a single gulp.

"What's wrong with this cat? Will she ever eat on her own?" I asked myself. Worries crept into my mind. Without a mother and siblings to show her how to eat, would she ever learn? With animals, I almost never quit trying, but this orphan tested even my patience. The situation was so grim I started to wonder if she had a brain disorder. I placed another sample of gruel on a plate and sat it in front of the hungry kitten. She refused it again. With my finger, I wiped some on her mouth. She screamed and rubbed her face on a nearby towel. In desperation, I pushed her mouth into the food and gently held her there. She struggled for 10 seconds or so, then miraculously focused on the food. Her eyes widened as she finally tasted the gruel.

"Slurp, slurp, slurp." I watched in amazement. Genny held her lips in a perfect circle and sucked the food down like she did with the syringe. As I continued to watch, she finished the rest of it, reminding me of a miniature vacuum cleaner. By the end of the day, she learned to lick and chew. Before bed, I placed a bowl of food in her box. For the first time in five weeks, Steve and I slept all night long.

"Genny," I cried again as my father smiled. She responded with baby mews – the kind that melt your heart. She stuck her paw out the front of the carrier. I opened the door and cuddled her in my arms. "Did you have fun with Grandma and Grandpa?"

Dad squinted and frowned. "I'm not so sure Bobbe wants to be a grandma to a cat, Kris. Better not mention that around her." I ignored him and continued to cuddle Genny. She nuzzled her face into my neck and purred and purred and purred. She had grown a lot in the two weeks she stayed with my folks. Her body reminded me of teenager's, big feet that look out of place with a little body.

"I keep forgetting to ask about the dog that was hit by the car. What happened to him?" Dad asked.

I explained that Cody had broken his hip. He had surgery a week later. His owner included a nice thank-you note with a check for his care. When Cody returned home, he searched for the other dog. After a few days, he stopped looking and seemed to resign himself to the fact that his buddy was gone. Tommy said it was heartbreaking to see him so depressed and planned to get Cody a new friend as soon as his leg healed.

While Allie and I worked on our one and only surgery of the day, Dad worked on installing a new doorbell. He settled in with the directions and a thermos of coffee before attempting the project. Allie made a home for Genny in the bottom cage in the treatment room. She gave her a litter box with low sides, a bowl of water and a plate of food. In the corner, she placed the carrier with her favorite blanket inside. Genny ate two tablespoons of food and then settled into her crate. Within minutes, her eyes closed, and she drifted off to sleep.

The doorbell dinged over and over again as Dad fiddled with the installation, but Genny slept through it all, her body twitching as she dreamed. Even her little stump moved. She seemed glad to be home.

As always, Dad needed parts not included in the doorbell kit. He entered the treatment room and spotted Genny in the lower cage. He frowned with displeasure. "You're not going to keep her in there are you? That's cruel."

"It's not cruel," I responded and removed the surgical cap from my head. Animals, especially youngsters, need a safe spot to call home. Setting her up in a cage and sticking to a routine will help her feel secure. I also explained that I needed to limit the amount of exercise she received because of the stump. The bone had nothing but skin covering it. I did not want Genny to damage the hairless end on our hard clinic floors. Dad looked the other way and shook his head. I knew he disagreed. I would have to keep a close eye on her when he was in the clinic.

He cleared his throat. "I also came back to tell you that you have a client up front." Allie removed her cap and fluffed her hair. Two minutes later, she returned, fuming.

"It's the family with the bird." She pulled out a step stool and placed it in front of the bank of cages. She stepped up and pulled down a small birdcage. The family wanted to keep the cage and toys so they could get another bird when they settled in South Carolina. Allie rolled her eyes. "They don't have room for the little bird, but they have room for the cage. People make me so mad."

Dad looked at me in disbelief. When I was young, we always took our dog with us on trips. I remember sitting in the cab of the truck with Duchess. I passed the time by dressing the German shepherd in bandanas and headbands. The good-natured dog put up with me for hours on end. Soon, my parents would head south to their home in Florida with their two dogs, Peeper and Louisa. Dad had never heard of a family abandoning their pet. To him, animals were part of the family.

I explained that moving is a common reason people give when surrendering their pets. One cause may be our societal view of pets as property. Some people think animals are a commodity that can be exchanged without consequence. They forget about the emotional distress the animal experiences. When it's relinquished, the poor pet feels abandoned by its family. The animal goes from sleeping on the bed with its people to a cage at a shelter with countless other homeless pets. If only people looked beyond themselves and considered their actions from the pet's point of view, this might not be an epidemic problem.

Dad stood for a minute with his lips pressed in a frown. He jingled the change in his pocket but did not speak. For the first time, Dad experienced my world as a veterinarian. He understood why my patience with people does not always match my unlimited patience with animals and why the work is both rewarding and depressing at the same time. He understood the horrible situation that many veterinarians find themselves in – adopt the pet or else. Now he knew why veterinarians and technicians have so many pets. It's hard to say no to an innocent victim, especially when it has an adorable face like Genny's.

CHAPTER 5

Allie Rescues a Cat

I arrived at the clinic late. Allie sat behind the counter with the phone wedged between her ear and shoulder. A small colorful bird ran back and forth across the counter, his nails clicking against the slick vinyl surface. At four inches tall, he was dwarfed by the pencil caddy. He stopped to chew on the business cards in a plastic holder, his colorful red beak shining bright against the white cards.

"Good morning, Romeo," I said, moving the card-holder out of his reach. "Let's save a few for the clients, OK?" Allie hung up the phone.

"What happened last night?" Allie asked without offering a greeting.

"I treated a Pomeranian for an allergic reaction." I extended my finger toward Romeo. He put his foot up and then changed his mind.

The poor Pomeranian could not breathe when she had arrived at the clinic, gasping, for each breath. Her swollen face reminded me of a beach ball. She could barely open her eyes. I injected her with diphenhydramine and steroids to calm the reaction and placed her in an oxygen chamber. Thirty minutes later, her face returned to its normal size. With the swelling gone, she breathed with ease. The little dog licked me when I sent her home.

Romeo walked over to the plant sitting in the corner, stood on his tiptoes and reached up with his red beak. He couldn't quite reach the leaves. He stretched even further, but the lowest leaf still hovered half an inch above his head. "Anything new this morning?" I asked.

"Spaatz's owner called and scheduled a recheck for next week. Your Dad called and said he'll bring the dogs with him when he comes to fix the doorbell." She took a deep breath. "And there's a stray cat in back." She shot a tentative glance my way.

On the way to work, Allie noticed a lump of fur lying in the road. She thought it was another roadkill. Many raccoons and skunks die around here when they try to cross the roads. Allie swerved to avoid the body. As the car sped by, the animal lifted its head. Those were not the ears of a wild animal. They were perfect little triangles of white. The lump was a kitten.

Allie clapped a hand over her mouth in horror and slammed on the brakes. She ran toward the kitten, hoping to rescue it before another car whizzed by. When she approached, the kitten lifted its head and meowed. Allie knew that rescuing an injured animal is risky. Fearful and in pain, many typically wonderful animals will bite the good Samaritans trying to help them.

Allie paused for a split second and looked down the road. Headlights glowed in the distance. Because she's a veterinary technician, and with the kitten in danger, she scooped it up and ran back onto the shoulder of the road. A minute later, a large supply truck rambled by. It would have finished off the kitten.

Back in the car, Allie placed the animal on the passenger seat and cranked up the heat. The poor little thing looked so small and emaciated. Allie lifted its tail and determined it was a boy. He purred all the way to the clinic, happy to be lying on a soft leather seat instead of hard pavement.

The bedraggled kitten allowed me to remove him from the hospital cage without a struggle. I laid him on the treatment table and watched his chest move. Breathing was work. Based on his size, I guessed his age somewhere around 10 weeks. Performing a physical exam on him reminded me of anatomy lab in veterinary school. I could feel all of the bones and internal organs easily beneath the skin. He had zero subcutaneous fat; his hip bones stuck out like a milk cow's. When I parted his oil-slicked fur, little black dots scattered. Fleas! I felt itchy again.

I started at his head and worked down to his tail. Our instructors drilled this methodical approach into us as interns. The attending docs were unmerciful if we deviated from the protocol. Through the years, it helped me discover many surprises and unlock several mysteries. In the exam room, I encourage owners to examine their pets, touching every part of their bodies. I give examples of how owners caught problems early and saved their pets' lives. I also tell the owners how touch reduces blood pressure, calming both humans and animals in the process.

Black debris filled both of the kitten's ears, making it difficult to visualize his eardrums. Probably ear mites, based on his condition. I collected a sample on a cotton swab for examination under the microscope. His green eyes sparkled in the light of the ophthalmoscope. Much to my surprise, his retinas looked great. I expected to find lesions due to poor nutrition.

Next, he permitted me to open his mouth for a full inspection of the teeth. Six adult incisors filled the space between the right and left canine teeth on both the upper and lower jaws. Right beside each fang, a second smaller tooth poked through the inflamed gingival tissue – his adult canines. He was teething. In cats, the adult canine teeth erupt at four to six months of age. Based on this dental examination, I now estimated his age at five months. He was much older than his size indicted. Baby teeth filled the rest of his mouth.

As a general rule, kittens weigh about 100 grams at birth and gain five to 10 grams a day. At five months, a normal kitten weighs between two- and three-and-a-half pounds. I stood staring at the scale in disbelief. Our little stray weighed in at a minuscule pound. His emaciation was far worse than I imagined. I found no palpable fat anywhere on his body. A wave of dread spread over me. Many animals in this condition die regardless of the course or duration of treatment.

As I listened to his heart, the tiny kitten purred. He seemed to soak up the attention, even from a vet. The purring made it tough to listen to his heart. I bent down and blew on his face. He stopped purring, looking at me with an annoyed expression. "Lub dub, lub dub, lub dub." The rate and rhythm sounded good. I did not hear a murmur.

"I'm sorry little purrbox, but I needed to listen to your heart." The kitten looked up at me for an instant before closing his eyes and purring again.

The next phase of the physical exam involved palpating his swollen abdomen. Both kidneys palpated normally or were "within normal limits," as I was trained to say. The urinary bladder felt small and soft through the abdominal wall. I squished gas through the intestines with my fingers. The intestines felt kind of "ropey" instead of the normal soft and doughy. Worms, I guessed. I finished the exam by feeling each of his legs. I did not find any fractures.

"What do you think, Dr. Nelson?" Allie asked as she walked into the treatment room. She stroked his dirty face as a look of concern spread across her own. "He's so small," she muttered.

I smiled but did not answer. Based on his rapid respiratory rate and pot-bellied appearance, I worried about feline infectious peritonitis. He could also have feline immunodeficiency virus or feline leukemia virus. If he tested negative for those three diseases, he might have a chance. If, that is, his internal organs weren't already damaged by the starvation. I felt a pit grow in my stomach. He needed every one of his nine lives to survive. He needed them all now.

Blood tubes with different colored tops, needles and a syringe appeared from beneath the table. Drawing blood from a cat can be done in a variety of ways, although it is usually a two- person job. Small veins on the inner aspect of the back legs work well for fractious cats, as these veins are far from the teeth. The technician holds the cat in a stretched position – on its side by the scruff of the neck, with the back legs extended. Another reason to use back legs for drawing blood is to reserve the veins on the front legs for intravenous catheters. The only drawback associated with using the veins on the back legs is size. They're small, limiting the rate at which blood flows into the syringe. Sometimes, clotting occurs before the sample can be mixed with anticoagulant.

A faster choice for drawing blood is to use one of the two large jugular veins on the neck. One person restrains the cat with its head up and front feet pulled down, usually over the end of a table. A second person draws the blood. Rubbing alcohol flattens down the hair, exposing the vein. The phlebotomist places her finger low on the cat's neck, blocking the flow of blood and causing the jugular to swell from the pooling blood. A quick poke later, the blood draw is over.

"He needs a name," Allie said as I positioned the kitten with his front feet over the end of the table for a jug stick. "What do you think we should call him?"

"I think you should wait until we know the results. I don't want to get attached to him if we have to euthanize."

Like most techs in these situations, Allie ignored my suggestion and offered a few names, all related to Star Trek. She loved the kitten already. Like other veterinary professionals, she dealt with serious disease by assuming the best until the worst actually occurred. Staffs name strays to bring them good luck. I knew she would clip his nails as well, another good-luck ritual in the veterinary profession.

"How about Kirk or McCoy?" she asked. "Or maybe Tribble ... that would be cute." None of the names she tried fit the scruffy little dirtball. My suggestion of Scruffy stuck by default since Allie could not settle on a superior alternative. Other than purring, the kitten was too weak to display any kind of personality. His filthy hair made it impossible to even tell the true color of his fur. Scruffy would have to do until we learned more about this tiny creature.

With the blood draw over, I needed to establish his feeding schedule. The biggest mistake people make with starving animals is feeding them too much, too soon. It's counterintuitive, but restraint is the key to prevent a condition called "re-feeding syndrome." Through the years, in both human and veterinary medicine, we have come to understand that individuals who gorge themselves after a period of prolonged starvation die, while those who gradually increase their caloric intake, live.

During starvation, organ function drops as the body shifts from metabolizing carbohydrates to using its own reserves of fat and protein for energy. Overfeeding a patient in this condition causes a precipitous drop in magnesium, potassium and phosphorous as well as overexpansion of the extracellular fluid volume. Death results from such complications as respiratory failure, heart problems, red-blood-cell destruction, generalized muscle weakness, coma and seizures.

To avoid this syndrome, patients should be treated with a high-fat, low-carbohydrate diet supplemented with potassium, magnesium and phosphorous. Even with careful monitoring, some patients cannot overcome the severe problems caused by starvation. Scruffy had long odds stacked against him.

"OK Allie, feed him two tablespoons of our critical-care diet." I looked at her sternly. "Only two." She nodded and placed two tablespoons on a small plate. Scruffy sniffed the food, froze for a second and dove in. He gulped it in four large mouthfuls. Some food oozed from the corners of his mouth. He licked the plate for a minute after all the food was gone, then looked up and begged for more.

"Sorry, bud, Dr. Nelson says only two," Allie responded. She sprayed him with flea spray, wrapped a towel around him and put him back in his cage. We didn't want fleas spreading to any other animals in the clinic. She placed two hot water bottles around him for extra warmth. Short of owning an incubator, it was the best we could do. The exhausted little guy closed his eyes, purred and drifted off to sleep. Hopefully, the nightmare of his ordeal would fade from his dreams.

CHAPTER 6

Bridget Lacerates Her Paw

Dad walked into the clinic with a triumphant look, holding up a plastic bag filled with parts. "What are you going to work on today, Gordy?" Allie asked.

"I'm going to finish the doorbell," my dad replied.

Allie raised her arms and danced in place. Without a doorbell, we didn't know when clients entered the building. Poor Allie ran from the treatment room to the lobby constantly. Her shins ached from running on the hard floor.

Dad smiled. He wanted the project finished just as badly as she did. My parents were eager to leave Minnesota before the snow flew. The surf and sand of Florida called. Most importantly, Dad's golf league started in two weeks.

By noon, a loud "ding, ding" rang out every time the front door opened. While he worked, his pups, Louisa and Peeper, stood vigil in the truck. Because of the cool weather, they could stay in the cab with the windows partially rolled down. A tall Lab mix, Louisa looked like a person sitting in the passenger seat, watching people come and go from the clinic with a smile on her face. A terrier mix, little Peeper stood on her back legs with her paws resting on the back of the seat. She could care less about people. She scanned the horizon for anything that moved. Her persistence paid off when she spotted a squirrel in the grassy area on the far side of the parking lot. A squirrel maniac, she pushed her snout through the open wing window and drank in the scent.

Dad and I walked down to the local Burger King for lunch. We stood in line surrounded by high school students wearing faded jeans and letter jackets. When it came time to pay, Dad pulled his wallet from his back pocket.

"I've got it, Dad," I told him. He looked surprised. "Just a little thank-you for all the work you have done at the clinic. I don't know what I would have done without you." He smiled and put away his wallet. Like all fathers, he typically paid for everything. Watching me pay for lunch filled him with pride. It was a small gesture, financially insignificant, but he reveled in the moment.

After lunch, Dad brought the girls in for their examinations. Louisa happily trotted into the clinic. Peeper took one step inside and tried to retreat to the safety of the truck. She knew from the smell where she was and did not like it. Dad picked her up and carried her into the treatment room. Coarse, wiry hair covered her body in large patches of black and white. Along the top of her body, the hair grew several inches longer than the rest, resulting in a bonafide mohawk. My mother hated it. She always brushed the longer hairs down against Peeper's body.

"Peeper has developed mild gingivitis, Dad." I lifted her lip and showed him the inflamed gums. "You need to brush her teeth, or I'll have to knock her out for a dental when you come back next spring." He looked dismayed at the prospect of having to brush the dog's teeth. "Other than that, she looks great." I patted her on the head. She turned away and looked at Dad.

"OK, Louisa, it's your turn." Louisa trotted over. My parents adopted her the summer before I started veterinary school. My mother always liked the The Sound of Music, so we named her Louisa. Her blond coat made her easy to spot. "Wheezy" grew into a gentle giant without a mean bone in her body. Her mission in life was to please the people around her.

"Sit," I ordered. Her rear end dropped to the ground. She brushed her tail back and forth on the floor. I taught her basic obedience while on vacation from veterinary school. She learned "sit," "down," "come" and "heel" in two weeks. The next summer, she learned to roll over for a treat. Sometimes, she rolled over four or five times in a row just to make sure she received the treat. As I knelt down to examine her, Wheezy lay down and flipped onto her back with her legs up in the air. She remained in this position for the entire examination.

"She looks good, too, Dad," I pronounced happily. I stood up and adjusted the stethoscope around my neck. "Be sure and keep them on the heartworm preventative while you are in Florida. Heartworm is a big problem down there." He nodded and jingled Wheezy's leash. She flipped onto her side and stared at Dad with her brown eyes. Peeper barked and circled in place. They loved to ride in the truck and were ready to roll.

"Well, Krissy, I'm going to take off if you don't need anything else. Your mother has a million things for me to do before we leave." He clipped the leash onto Louisa's collar and hoisted Peeper onto his shoulder.

"Have a safe trip and call me when you arrive," I said. I hugged him first and then the two dogs. "And remember to brush their teeth." He did not acknowledge my comment. I made a mental note to tell my mother the next time we spoke.

The rest of the day passed uneventfully. At 5, Allie flew out the door. Her favorite band was playing at a bar near her apartment, and she needed time to get ready. At 6, I turned on the answering machine and flipped on my pager. The clinic had not done much revenue for the day. With all the start-up costs and my car on the line with the bank, I needed business to pick up before our savings ran out. As I slipped the pager in my pocket, it started to buzz. Maybe this would make up for the slow day.

"Hello, Kris, this is Sally Smith," said the voice on the phone. "Sorry to bother you, but I think Bridget needs stitches."

Twenty minutes later, a beautiful Irish setter entered the clinic wearing a white bandage soaked with blood on her right front paw. The entourage included Sally, her husband, Joe and their young son, Jason. Sally and Joe were avid outdoor enthusiasts who loved hunting birds. In their living room, a prize taxidermy specimen hung over the TV. During the holidays, Sally hung lights around the stuffed pheasant and tied a bright red ribbon around its neck. Joe preferred the bird without the accessories.

Every year, the family hunted grouse and pheasant in northern Minnesota. Bridget combed the countryside in search of prey with a determination second to none. She would ford any stream or jump through the roughest brush in search of a bird. When she found one, she froze in place with her nose pointed at the bird and front foot off the ground. Her body formed a mahogany-colored arrow. On command, she rushed forward and flushed the birds for her owners. If they missed, she gave them a dirty look. Bridget held Sally and Joe to the same high standard she expected of herself.

About two months before the season opened, Joe started to condition Bridget for the rigors of hunting. After work, the two played fetch in the backyard. As her fitness improved, Joe lengthened the sessions. They were almost finished with the evening workout when Bridget stopped in the middle of a retrieve and held up her paw. Blood dripped to the ground. Joe immediately got Sally, who wrapped the foot to control the bleeding and called me.

I removed the bloodsoaked bandage, not knowing what to expect. Bridget rested quietly on the floor with her head in Joe's lap. Blood oozed from the central pad of her foot. A deep laceration ran from one side to the other.

"What do you think?" Sally asked.

"You were right," I replied. "This definitely needs stitches."

"Will she be able to hunt?" Joe asked. It was the first question any serious hunter would ask, and Joe was serious about hunting.

The family was planning a special trip to Wisconsin with friends in addition to its usual outings in Minnesota. Joe bought Bridget a neoprene vest for the trip just to keep his girl warm in the field.

I pondered Joe's question. Pad injuries are difficult to treat. It takes a long time for the thick protective surface of the pad to regenerate. A laceration like this could take months to heal because of the constant wear and tear when the dog walked or ran. She could be on the injured reserve list for the entire season.

"How long before you leave?' I asked.

"About two weeks," Joe answered. Deep furrows appeared in his forehead. He exchanged a nervous glance with Sally. That was not the answer I hoped for. A month maybe, but two weeks ... her chances of hunting were slim to none.

"I'm not sure this will heal by then, Joe. The stitches will still be in." He continued to stroke her head without making a sound. He looked deflated. The thought of going without Bridget was too much. "But maybe we can figure out a way to bandage the foot that will still allow her to go," I added.

I repaired the wound with heavy-duty nylon suture and covered it with a sturdy wrap. Bridget felt better with the pain medicine in her system, but she hated the bandage. She shook her paw and held it off the floor. With encouragement, she put it on the tile and walked with an exaggerated limp. She took a few steps, then looked up at Joe for help.

"Sorry, Bridget," he said. "You're going to have to get used to that." She limped over to Sally for a second opinion.

"No, I'm not going to take it off either. For goodness sake, these pets are just like children." She chuckled. "Dad said no, so she tried mom. Honestly Bridget, you are too smart."

I showed Sally and Joe how to check Bridget's toes for swelling. If the bandage constricted her leg, her foot would swell. The middle toes would separate, and the bandage would have to be removed. If Bridget licked or chewed the bandage, she would have to wear the dreaded e-collar. Finally, I explained how bandages tighten up with moisture.

Bridget tried to lick my face as I placed a plastic bag over her bandage. Animals are so forgiving. I always marvel at how they forgive and forget. I scratched her back to reward her.

When the Smith's van left the parking lot, I prepared to leave the clinic. Before I left, I checked on Genny. She lay on her back at the front of her cage playing with a small plastic ball. The bell inside jingled when she kicked it with her front feet. I stuck my finger through the bars and rubbed her tummy.

Next, I looked into Scruffy's cage. He lay on a water heating pad with his entire body wrapped in blankets, except for his head. His eyes were half open, half closed. They looked dull, almost glazed over. I watched the blankets for movement. Seconds ticked by ... I did not see his chest move.

"Scruffy! Scruffy!" I called. The kitten did not respond. I dropped my bag on the floor. The noise startled Genny, and her plastic ball rattled to the floor as she scurried for the safety of her carrier.

I opened the latch to Scruffy's cage and pulled back the blankets. Scruffy continued to lie on his side without moving. I felt my heart in my throat as I placed my fingers around his chest. Nothing, I felt nothing. When I repositioned my fingers again, I felt his heart beating in a slow regular rhythm. A second later, he took a deep breath.

"Scruffy, don't scare me like that." I rubbed my finger along his chin. The kitten opened his eyes for a second and then closed them again. He looked so pathetic. I replaced the blankets around his body and placed some lube in both of his eyes before slowly closing the cage door. A feeling of dread crept over me. "Bye, Scruffy," I said, my voice cracking as I spoke. "I hope I see you tomorrow."

CHAPTER 7

Scruffy Fights for Life

G ray clouds loomed overhead as I drove to the clinic. A sharp chill filled the air, a precursor of weather to come. Beautiful gold and red leaves skittered across the road. I shivered and readjusted the vent. October in Minnesota is a transitional month. Some days are warm with beautiful puffy clouds filling the sky while others are cold and gray, informing all who live in the "Land of 10,000 Lakes" that winter approaches.

"Hello, how are you?" Bongo greeted my arrival at the clinic without understanding the words. Feathers ruffled in the other cages. Usually, I uncover the birds, put my coat and bag in the office and check the answering machine. Today I marched straight into the back ignoring Bongo's greeting and Windsor's wolf whistle. All night long, I tossed and turned, unable to sleep because of Scruffy. Would he survive? I feared our help came too late to save him.

In the treatment room, Scruffy was in the exact position I left him the night before. "Scruffy! Scruffy!" I called his name. Nothing happened. He did not move. I opened the door to his cage and pushed it aside with urgency. The door swung into the next cage with a bang. Scruffy flinched and opened his eyes.

His lab results looked good. The tests did not detect antibodies for feline leukemia, feline infectious peritonitis or feline immunodeficiency virus. So far, his electrolytes registered in the normal range, albeit at the low end. With feeding, the values would decrease even further as the electrolytes shifted from the blood back into the cells. By anticipating this shift, we hoped to catch it early before any life-threatening complications occurred.

For several days, Scruffy slept under a pile of blankets. Hot water circulated in a rubber heating mat, providing warmth since he could not sustain his own body temperature. I never use a standard electric heating pad because of the potential to burn the patient and the possibility of electrocution. Allie hand fed and watered him several times a day. He urinated in bed right where he lay. He was too weak to turn himself over, let alone walk to the litter box. Sometimes, the movement of his chest was the only clue he was still alive.

We treated his ear mites and intestinal worms. Bathing would have to wait until his condition improved. Right now, eating and drinking exhausted the little fellow. He spent virtually the entire day sleeping. An aura of immense sadness surrounded the bedraggled kitten as he struggled to survive.

A week later, Allie and I worked on an emergency in the treatment room. An Amazon parrot just like Bongo broke a blood feather in her wing. The owner returned home to find blood dripping from her bright green parrot and spattered all over the cage. She rushed her in for emergency care. Large drops of burgundy blood fell from the bird's wing and pooled on the bottom of the carrier.

We had to act fast because birds can easily die from this condition. I estimated her weight at 500 grams, which meant she could safely loose about five milliliters or one teaspoon of blood! From the owner's description and the amount of blood pooled on the newspaper, she might already have exceeded that limit.

I reached into the carrier, giving the command "step up!"

Instead of lifting a foot to my hand, the bird lunged at me with a gaping beak.

"Bummer," I muttered. Using a towel, I thrust my now protected hand into the carrier. I grabbed the backside of the bird's head with my fingers on each side of her lower jaw. In this position, I controlled the powerful beak. I folded the wings against her body before removing her from the travel crate.

"Here you go, Allie." Holding birds looks a lot easier than it is. The holder must restrain the bird's beak, wings and nails to prevent injury to the medical staff as well as the bird. Because birds do not have a diaphragm, the chest wall must move during each breath. If the towel is wrapped too tight, or if pressure is put on the chest, the bird will suffocate. Allie slipped her fingers behind mine and positioned the bird against her chest.

I removed the towel from the affected wing and extended it away from her body. Blood oozed from the base of the third flight feather. New feathers grow from a feather follicle. A rich supply of blood extends up the shaft, giving the area a blue, fleshy appearance. When the feather matures, the blood supply recedes, leaving the firm white shaft or spine that is commonly recognized. If traumatized, these immature feathers called blood feathers may bleed insidiously. To stop it, the offending feather must be removed.

With Allie holding the wing in a stretched position, I placed the jaws of a hemostat around the feather and held the base of the wing in my other hand. With slow, steady traction, the feather came out all in one piece. Blood oozed from the hole left behind.

"Good job, Kris," Allie said, repositioning the bird in her arms. If proper technique is not used, the follicle can be damaged, preventing further feather growth. Worse yet, the wing itself might fracture. I applied pressure to the follicle for a minute before closing it with a drop of tissue adhesive. We would observe her for a few hours before sending her home.

As Allie put the bird back in her carrier, a loud crash followed by a thud emanated from Scruffy's cage. Litter flew through the front bars of the stainless-steel cage and landed on the floor. Scruffy lay in his litter box, all four feet splayed in different directions. Bits of litter stuck to his face and whiskers. He looked up and meowed pitifully.

"Good job, buddy!" I cheered.

"A for effort," Allie echoed. We could hardly contain our excitement and relief. During his first trip to the box, he lifted three feet over the edge, but ran into trouble with the fourth. With a little help, he postured and urinated in the box. When he finished, he closed his eyes and purred. Allie beamed with joy. "I think he's going to make it, Dr. Nelson." We stood outside his cage in silence, overcome with emotion. I nodded and blinked back tears. I live for these moments. The joy of pulling a critical animal back from the brink of death is priceless.

Sadly, our celebration was brief. The doorbell rang, announcing that Spaatz was here for his recheck. Allie left to check him in while I called the bird's owner with an update. With the bleeding stopped, the bird looked much better.

Since our last visit, Bob Williams instilled four drops of medicine in Spaatz's ear each day. He did so whether Spaatz wanted it or not. He caught the handsome tuxedo and wrapped him in a blanket for the treatment. This did nothing to improve the cat's mood. Long red scratches covered the man's arms. Evidently, Spaatz hid under the bed during the day, only coming out when Bob slept.

Before I even opened the carrier, Spaatz started to hiss. He knew what was coming. With the door open, the hisses morphed into a growl. Their deep and rumbling nature warned us that Spaatz was really angry, angry at us for his visit to the clinic, angry at his owner for bringing him in, angry at life in general. I held the carrier with the open door facing down to the table. A young vet might try to reach in and show the cat who was boss. I had too much experience for that. Spaatz slid out. He glared at me with bright green eyes, his hair on end.

While I distracted him, Allie grabbed the scruff of his neck with one hand and flattened him onto the table. I inserted the otoscope cone and hoped for the best. Healthy pink mucosa replaced the inflamed mess I saw before. Bob's hard work had paid off. The mites were gone. I opened the door to the carrier, and Allie turned Spaatz around. Once he saw the open door, the angry cat ran in hissing all the way.

"Good news, Bob," I smiled. "His ears look great except for one large clump of wax on his right eardrum." Bob breathed a sigh of relief. Spaatz swiped at my fingers as I closed the carrier door. I felt a breeze across my knuckles.

"That's great news," he said. He pointed to an inflamed area on his right wrist. The wound occurred this morning when he put Spaatz in the crate. "He won't let me touch him anymore because he thinks I'm going to put medicine in his ear." He looked into the carrier, and Spaatz hissed. Bob became serious. "Will he ever love me again, Dr. Nelson?"

"Absolutely!" I put my hand on his shoulder. "He's just a little ticked off right now, but he'll get over it." I explained how cats sometimes associate people with negative events even when they're over. "For example, let's say a mean dog cornered Spaatz. Before the dog attacked, you rescued him. He should be grateful, right?" Bob nodded. "But that's not always how it works. He might associate you with the scary dog and hiss." I assured Bob that once Spaatz realized the treatments were over, he would become a loving companion again. But for now, Mr. Attitude would need to stay with us for an ear flush.

Allie placed the carrier in the lower cage next to Genny's home, giving Spaatz a litter pan and blanket. With the cage arranged, she opened the carrier's door. Spaatz growled from within. Genny jumped down from her cage and ran out of the room. "Cut it out," Allie ordered as she closed the cage door. "You're scaring Genny."

Spaatz continued to growl and hiss whenever anyone passed his cage. We dreaded working with him. I covered his carrier with a towel and closed Spaatz inside before transferring him to the table. From the back room Allie retrieved a plastic anesthesia chamber that resembled an aquarium. Because we couldn't touch Spaatz without risking our lives, we planned to box him down in the chamber.

Allie unclamped the chamber lid and nodded. I gingerly opened the door to his carrier with a towel wrapped around my hand for protection. Next, I slowly inverted the carrier over the chamber. But Spaatz remembered this maneuver from before, braced his body against the sides and hissed.

Allie bent over and strained to look up into the carrier. "He's not coming out," Allie said. Spaatz assumed a spread-eagle position inside. He dug into the edges of the carrier with his claws and growled.

"Let me give him a little help." I rocked the carrier until I felt him move. He lost his toehold and slipped out into the chamber. Allie covered it before he could escape. She hooked the hose from the anesthesia machine to a fitting on the chamber and turned the dial to high. Spaatz wiggled his nose when he smelled the anesthetic gas mixed with oxygen and spun around the chamber, clawing and digging to get out.

"Stop fighting it," Allie encouraged the cat. "When you wake up, the nightmare will be over." Spaatz ignored her. He continued to fight and claw, but he was no match for the isoflurane. With every breath, he became more and more sleepy. Finally, he lay quietly in the chamber.

"Do you think he's ready, Dr. Nelson?" Allie asked.

"Let me check before you take the lid off. I don't want to take any chances," I replied. I tilted the chamber. Spaatz slid from one end to the other without resistance. He was out. The worst part was over, and no one, including Spaatz, got hurt. It was a small victory, but those count, too.

With Spaatz asleep, we removed him from the chamber and passed a tracheal tube down his throat. Two minutes later, he lay on the table surrounded by beeping monitors. Allie placed a half-inch of lube in both of his eyes to protect them from drying out. I put a towel under his head and thrust an otoscope cone down his ear.

After dealing with Spaatz' attitude, the ear flush itself was a piece of cake. We flushed out the ball of wax with a long catheter. He returned to his cage with spotless ears and a dose of pain medicine. We propped his head up on towels to decrease the amount of swelling. He winked his eyes and for the first time, I heard him purr.

"What's next on the agenda, Allie?" I asked as I washed my hands at the surgical prep sink.

"Bridget Smith will be here soon to recheck her foot," she answered. "After that, I thought I would give Scruffy a bath."

With only a week to go before the big hunting trip, Bridget's paw took a turn for the worse. I removed the bandage, horrified by what I saw. The surface of her pad had softened up and begun to slough. The normally calloused surface was pliable. Worse, the sutures had fallen out. They cut through the abnormal tissue like it was butter. Large chunks of her central pad fell off, and the remaining tissue looked like raw hamburger. Nothing would hold the laceration together now. I decided to leave it open for few days under a protective bandage. If things went well, perhaps I could try to close it again in a couple of days. The hunting trip looked highly unlikely for Bridget.

As soon as Bridget left the clinic, Allie carried Scruffy to the kennel and gently placed him in the empty bathtub. The large tub dwarfed his small body. He stood motionless, surveying the new surroundings. Across from the tub, he heard the washer rock back and forth as it cleaned a load of towels. The strange noises intrigued him. Bottles of shampoo and various flea and tick dips filled the corners of the tub. He stood up on his hind legs and sniffed the bottles.

While the water warmed, Scruffy explored the other end of the bathtub, away from the faucet. His eyes were huge. When the temperature reached perfection, Allie held the back of his neck with one hand and sprayed water over him with the other. Scruffy arched his back and meowed pathetically. A look of disdain spread over his face. He held up one paw at a time and shook the water from it.

"What's wrong, Scruff?" Allie teased. "Don't you like your bath?" Scruffy stared into her eyes and meowed again. Before lathering him in flea shampoo, she protected his eyes with ointment. He stood on his back legs with both front feet resting on the side of the tub and continued to shake his paws. Water flew in all directions. Dark wet spots dotted Allie's scrubs.

Poor Scruffy looked like a skinny drowned rat. He continued to meow forlornly, all the while looking for an escape route. Genny hopped into the room to see what all the fuss was about. She stood below the tub, looking up at the bedraggled kitten. Both were about the same age, yet Genny – three legs and all – was much bigger.

"You want to be next, Genevieve?" Allie teased. Genny promptly turned and left.

After a 10-minute soak, Allie rinsed the shampoo from Scruffy. His meows increased in intensity the closer the spray came to his face. He had been a good sport in the beginning, but enough was enough. When Allie momentarily loosened her grip, he jumped over the side. She caught him in midair, returning him to the dreaded bathtub. Like I said, you have to be quick in this profession.

Wrapped in a towel with only his face showing, Scruffy continued to meow. "Meeeeoooowww, meeeeoooowww." His cries formed a staccato rhythm as Allie toweled him off. She smiled and planted a kiss on his forehead. After a quick blow dry, the bath was over. Scruffy returned to his cage, exhausted but clean. He snuggled into a thick blanket and drifted off to sleep.

With the oil and dirt gone, Scruffy's true colors came to life. He was a gorgeous specimen. Short white fur that felt like a fine cashmere sweater, soft and thick, covered most of his body. Patches of charcoal grey adorned his face, back and tail. It looked like someone sponge-painted these blocks of color along his dorsal line. His nose and pads were pink with a few black spots. He looked great except for the frayed whiskers sticking out in unusual directions on his face.

Allie walked into the office, rubbing lotion onto her hands. "Scruffy is done," she announced proudly. "Let's get Genny's last set of vaccinations done before the afternoon appointments start." I nodded and followed her into the treatment room. Genny sat in front of the bank of cages, tormenting the animals inside. She so wickedly loved to do this. She held her stump off the floor. A thick callus now covered the end.

"Come here, little princess." I scooped her into my arms. "It's your turn." Genny cried and fought to escape. As a little kitten, Genny would lie in my arms for hours. She purred and kneaded my stomach as she nursed on my finger. Now, as a five-month-old teenager, she hated being held and exuded the most bloodcurdling sound whenever an insignificant human tried it.

"Here's her last vaccination, feline leukemia," Allie informed me. She placed a syringe filled with pink fluid on the table. "I'll take the Princess." Allie held her arms out toward Genny.

"Don't you want to give her the shot?" I asked, still holding Genny.

"No, I don't want her to hate me."

"But it's OK for her to hate me?" I asked with a smile. Allie ignored my question. I obediently handed Genny to her. Allie laid her on the table, holding the scruff of her neck with one hand and her one normal back leg with the other. While Allie blew into her face, I popped the needle beneath the skin on her stump leg and injected the vaccine.

"See, it wasn't so bad, Miss Genevieve," I cooed. Genny's eyes narrowed, and she swished her tail back and forth. She was not pleased. She lay on the table and licked the injection site, her tail still swishing. She was mad with a capital M.

Allie, still with a firm grip on the cat, bent over and whispered, "Just remember Genny, it was her, not me."

CHAPTER 8

Owner's Intuition

We only had one appointment scheduled for the entire afternoon. A cat named Max was having accidents in the house. While his owner Joyce Segal, got ready for work, Max jumped into the sink, postured and urinated right in front of her. At the end of his stream, he produced a few drops of blood-tinged urine.

A year ago, Joyce found him lying in the litter box, straining to urinate. She rushed him to the emergency clinic for care. The veterinarian felt his abdomen and made the diagnosis. Max had feline urinary syndrome (FUS). Minerals in his urine precipitated out of solution and formed small pieces of grit in his bladder. When he urinated, the grit clogged his urethra. The cat could not urinate, and his pain seemed unbearable. The veterinarian knocked Max out, passed a urethral catheter and drained his bladder. The urine looked like tomato soup as it flowed into a collection bag. After three days of treatment, and being tethered to a bag, he went home. He now passed yellow urine with ease.

The large orange cat sat on the table as his owner recounted his medical history. His magnificent markings caught my eye. Beautiful swirls of deep rust-colored fur danced across his sides. The swirls formed a perfect M on his forehead like Genny, the final exclamation point for this classic tabby. He thumped his tail as cats do when annoyed. When Joyce finished speaking, he stood up, walked to the end of the table and urinated right in front of us.

A look of horror spread across Joyce's face. She grabbed a tissue from her leather purse. "Don't clean it up," I instructed. Her hand froze in mid-air, and she shot me a quizzical glance. I retrieved a syringe from the cabinet drawer and aspirated the urine off the table-top. I needed to analyze it for crystals. Since Max provided a sample, we would not have to stick him.

While Allie studied the urine, I examined Max. His bladder felt empty and soft.

"Good news, Joyce," I announced. "He's not blocked. You caught it before it became an emergency."

A look of relief spread over Joyce's face. "That's the first thing that's gone right all day." She smiled but did not elaborate. "Why did this happen?"

I needed to do a little detective work before I could answer. Once Max received the FUS diagnosis, he started on a special diet to dissolve crystals in his urinary tract, then switched to a maintenance diet to keep any more from forming. Logically, the maintenance diet contains a higher amount of salt to increase water consumption. It also has reduced amounts of the minerals that form crystals.

Even so, some cats require distilled water to keep the problem in check. I have also observed that cats who suffer from chronic upper respiratory infections seem to have more recurrence than those who do not. I asked Joyce about his food and water. She reported that Max only ate a special diet.

"Do you remember the name?" I continued to probe. Unfortunately, she couldn't come up with the exact name. I listed a few, hoping to jog her memory.

"I used to feed him food that I purchased from the vet," she replied. "But he gained a lot of weight, so I switched him to another brand one month ago." She picked it up at the grocery store. It was cheaper and more convenient than making a trip to the clinic.

"Well, that's the problem," I replied. "Only the prescription diets are formulated to prevent the crystals from forming. The food is actually a treatment, which is why you have to purchase it from a veterinarian."

"But the package said it was good for urinary health," she countered.

I wish I had a dollar for every time I heard that statement. I could buy an incubator and still have money left over. Many brands of commercial cat food recently added this language to their packaging. Typically, these diets contain reduced levels of magnesium and ash to discourage crystal formation. But they do not contain acidifiers and all the other modifications needed to fully treat this condition. Sometimes marketing and medicine make poor bedfellows. The language confused people into buying the wrong food.

When Joyce realized her mistake, she placed her hand on her head and rubbed her temple. "I thought I was doing the right thing for Max," she whispered.

"Don't feel bad. I've seen many other people do the same thing." It was too bad for Max, though. He could have been spared a lot of discomfort. From her perspective, the vet bills would now exhaust the savings in food and then some. I made a note in Max's record. "Also, I want him to drink as much water as possible to flush out his bladder."

"He likes to sit in the sink and catch drips from the faucet," Joyce said.

"Great, let him do that several times a day." I picked up his record and got ready to leave the room. Joyce promised to never change his food again without prior consultation.

While I worked with Max, a woman arrived at the clinic with Sadie, her cocker spaniel. Paula Anderson found her beloved pet huddled in the corner when she returned from work. Small puddles

of foam surrounded her. The poor dog moaned and gagged when
Paula patted her abdomen. More white foam dripped from her
mouth. Sadie's regular vet could not see her. They recommended
going to the emergency clinic when they opened at 6 p.m., but
Paula didn't think Sadie could wait. She remembered our sign for
the Minnesota Veterinary Center and brought the dog here.

From the history and clinical signs, I suspected a condition
called bloat. The stomach fills with gas or food until it can no
longer empty. As more pressure builds, the stomach stretches to its
limit. Blood flow through the body is interrupted. If the stomach
is not decompressed quickly, shock develops. In the worst-case sce-
nario, the stomach actually twists on itself. These patients require
emergency surgery to reposition the stomach before the tissue dies.

As I examined Sadie, her buddy, Maggie, paced around the
room. The vizsla stopped every few steps to look up at Sadie. White
foam continued to fall from Sadie's mouth. I wiped it away and
pushed my finger-tip into her gum, just above the big canine tooth
on the left side. The pale pink gum blanched white and stayed that
way for over two seconds. I ran my hand down the inside of her
back leg until I felt the femoral artery pulse beneath my fingers. It
was much weaker than I expected. With the stethoscope on her
chest, I counted heartbeats and breaths. Both were elevated.

Next, I placed my hands on her abdomen. Most bloats occur in
large or giant-breed dogs because they simply have more room in
their abdomens than they need for their stomachs. While bloats
may occur in any breed, I had never seen one in a cocker spaniel.
Sadie's abdomen felt hard beneath my fingers. She moaned when
I tried to palpate her stomach. I stopped immediately and patted
her head.

"I'm glad you brought her right in, Ms. Anderson."

"Please, call me Paula."

"I think she's bloated. It's unusual in small dogs like Sadie, but
her signs are classic. We need to take an X-ray of her abdomen to
confirm the diagnosis."

Paula's lower lip quivered. "Is it fatal?" Her voice cracked as she spoke.

Her response surprised me. Perhaps I had not been as attentive to her nonverbal clues as I should have been. I tried to be more supportive and explained that while bloat can be fatal, most patients survive. The key is early diagnosis and treatment. We would start Sadie on fluids right away. If it was a simple bloat, I would pass a tube to relieve the pressure. If the stomach was twisted, she would need surgery.

I paused to let Paula absorb my words. Tears welled up in her eyes. She hugged Sadie then backed away from the table. Maggie put her front paws on Paula's knee. The sandy colored dog studied her owner's face for a minute before looking back at Sadie.

I wrapped Sadie in my arms to carry her to the treatment room. She moaned in pain.

A fresh bag of fluids hung from the I.V. stand in the treatment room. Allie clipped the dog's leg, disinfected it with iodine and placed the catheter. In less than two minutes, fluids dripped into Sadie's vein. The sickly pale pink color of her gums blossomed into a deeper hue of pink. Now it was time for an X-ray.

I carried Sadie through the kennel into the radiology suite. Allie pushed the I.V. pole and fluids behind us. We suited up in our colorful blue thyroid collars and lead-lined aprons, the heavy protective garments weighing us down. We lay Sadie on her side for the first film and on her back for the second. Allie slipped off her lead apron and headed to the darkroom with two cassettes in hand. Still clad in protective gear, I sat on the radiology table with Sadie until she returned.

"OK, both films are in the processor. It shouldn't be long now." Allie pulled out a large storage folder and wrote "Sadie Anderson" on the patient line. Next, she pulled a warm towel out of the dryer and wrapped it around the dog. The room-temperature fluids made her shiver. As I put my arm around her for added warmth, her blond fur felt like silk.

Cocker spaniels express so many emotions with their eyes. Sadie looked at me with her big brown eyes and begged for help. Her abdomen had grown larger in the short time she'd been in the clinic. She fidgeted back and forth on her front feet. The pain must have been unbearable.

The first film landed on the tray with a thud. Allie walked into the radiology suite, holding the film above her head. She used the overhead lights to illuminate it. I watched her eyes widen as she focused. "Whew, she's bloated all right." She handed the film to me. I snapped it in place on the view box.

"Wow!" I gasped at the size of Sadie's stomach. Never in my short career had I seen such a big stomach in this size dog. "We need to decompress her right away," I explained to Allie. In the center of the X-ray, a large black-colored circle filled most of the area underneath Sadie's ribs. Allie joined me at the viewer with Sadie in her arms. I scanned the film, looking for additional problems. The stomach did not appear twisted, and I found no obvious masses that might initially have caused the bloat. "I'll talk to Paula and get permission to knock her out."

Paula assented without hesitation. Allie and I worked quickly. We anesthetized Sadie and placed a trach tube down her airway. When she reached a good plane of anesthesia, Allie rolled Sadie on her side. I threaded a clear plastic tube down her esophagus; the tip stopped as it hit the stomach. I pushed with a little more force, but the tube would not budge. The distended stomach pinched the cardiac sphincter closed. It felt like the tube hit a brick wall.

I cleaned the free end of the stomach tube with alcohol on a gauze pad, inhaled deeply and placed my mouth around the tube. While I blew through one end, I pushed the other end down Sadie's throat with gentle force. It's a delicate, though unsightly, procedure. If I used too much force, the tube might rupture Sadie's esophagus or stomach. I twisted the tube to help it pass through the cardiac sphincter, but the tube would not budge. Beads of sweat formed under my bangs. I drew in another big breath and pushed on the tube as I blew into it with all my might.

Suddenly, I felt a pop. I removed my lips from the tube just in time to avoid a rush of gas! My bangs flew up into the air, and the smell of dog food filled the room. "Whew." I held the tube away from my face. It smelled like a frat house after a long weekend. "I always hate that part." Allie laughed.

For 10 minutes we flushed clean water into Sadie's stomach, rolled her around and then pumped the water out. At first, the brown-colored water contained dog food. The round pieces barely fit through the diameter of the stomach tube. By the end, the water ran clear.

At this point, with Sadie's stomach empty, we repositioned her body with her head hanging over the side of the table. I eased out the tube. Water and saliva dripped from Sadie's mouth and stuck in her beard. I held the tube over a drain and let the remaining contents run out. Allie wiped the dog's mouth and lifted her lip. The gums looked great. When Allie pressed them, the tissue blanched for a split second, then returned to pink. We kept her in this position for several minutes to prevent fluid from dripping down into her lungs. Aspiration pneumonia was the last thing this dog (or we) needed to combat.

While we waited for all the fluid to clear, I noticed Sadie's coat. The beautiful blond color reminded me of an oat field before harvest. Her long upper eyelashes looked fake, and her nails were trimmed and buffed to a smooth finish. What impressed me most was the cleanliness of her ears. Not a speck of wax anywhere. She looked like she stepped out of the show ring. This was obviously a well-beloved member of the family.

"Well groomed, isn't she?" Allie commented as she returned to the room. "This owner really takes good care of her. I wish every owner was like her." I nodded in response. With those big floppy ears, cocker spaniels require constant care ... weekly ear flushes and baths in addition to regular grooming. It's a huge responsibility – one many people do not fully appreciate.

After we cleaned up, I brought Paula back to the treatment

room. Allie wrapped Sadie in a blanket and placed a heating pad below her. She even sprayed the room with air freshener to mask the smell of partially digested dog food.

"She did just great," I informed the anxious owner. Paula bent over Sadie and hugged her. Maggie stood on her hind legs with her nose high in the air. She strained to look at her buddy, resting her front legs on the table. Her beautiful vizsla face lit up when she smelled her friend.

"Dr. Nelson, the post films are up." Allie slid them onto the viewer and turned on the light. I studied them while Paula petted her beloved companion, who shivered beneath the blankets.

"Why is she doing that?" Paula asked, concerned.

"She's cold from the anesthesia and the fluids," Allie answered. "While they're under, the body can't regulate its temperature." She pulled up a corner of the blanket. A green pad attached to a long plastic tube lay between Sadie and the table. Hot water circulated through the pump, into the water channels of the pad and then back to the pump for reheating.

"Good news, Paula." I turned to look at her. "I don't see any masses or other abnormalities."

Although Paula was happy, she wondered aloud why Sadie bloated in the first place? From the amount of food in her stomach, I guessed that Sadie ate too much and then drank a substantial amount of water. The kibble expanded in her stomach and caused the bloat.

Paula bent over Sadie and hugged her again. "Maggie would be lost without her," she stated. Maggie's ears perked up when she heard her name. "These two are inseparable."

Sadie started to cough and gag on the trach tube. Allie deflated the cuff, untied it from Sadie's upper jaw and held it by the end. When Sadie swallowed, she removed it from her throat and tossed it in the sink. Sadie coughed several times to clear her throat, opened her eyes and lifted her head off the table. With her tongue lolling to the side, she looked drunk. Paula giggled.

Allie brought a folding chair and placed it beside the table. Paula sat with her arms around Sadie while she recovered. Maggie sat beside the chair, facing the bank of cages behind the table, staring at Scruffy. During Sadie's treatment, he sat in the back of his cage grooming his coat after the bath. Satisfied with its condition, he walked back and forth along the front of the cage. He rubbed on the bars and purred. Maggie stared at the cat, unable to take her eyes off him.

"What's wrong with that cat?" Paula asked.

"He's a stray who needs a home," Allie answered with a big smile on her face. She winked at Paula. "I think he would make a great addition to your family." Paula started to laugh. She knew a sales job when she saw one. She held up her hands and shook her head.

"Two hands, two dogs ... that's my limit." Her face turned serious for a few seconds as she looked at Sadie. "Thanks to your wonderful care, I'm still at my limit."

"Well, if you know anyone who wants a cat, please tell them about Scruffy. We will vaccinate and neuter him for free," I said.

Feeling neglected, Sadie raised her paw and placed it on Paula's arm. When Paula looked at her, the dog uttered one sharp yip.

"What does she want?" Allie asked.

"That means she's ready to go." Tears flowed down Paula's cheeks. "She's back to normal." She buried her head in Sadie's fur. "My baby is back to normal."

CHAPTER 9

Nasty Animals

"Caution," Allie warned as she handed me a medical record. She stared at me for five seconds to make the point. "Be careful with this one, Kris." I nodded. Aggressive animals present the most dangerous aspect of veterinary medicine. In addition to physical trauma, I always worry about infection. One of my friends developed osteomyelitis from a cat bite. The infection in the bones of her knuckle required intravenous antibiotics and a hospital stay. She eventually had the joint fused to alleviate pain.

"Hello, I'm Dr. Nelson," I said entering the room. My canine patient reclined on the table. Thick fur masked her eyes. I could only discern a jet-black nose beneath the hair.

"Hello, Dr. Nelson, I'm Ed Allen, and this is Precious." He petted her head. "She's a real brat, so be careful." I appreciated his honesty. Ed adopted Precious when she was a puppy. He loved the little furball too much and spoiled her rotten. When the Lhasa apso turned a year old, Precious decided she ruled the roost, not her owner. She spent her life on the furniture, not on the floor like lesser dogs. If anyone tried to sit beside Ed on the couch, she growled. Precious also slept right in the middle of the bed while Ed clung to the edges. If he tried to move the feisty dog over, Precious growled and showed her teeth. She was a furry bully.

"So what is Precious in for today?" I asked.

"Well, the groomer put a bow on her, and she won't let me remove it." He pointed to a tangle of hair on the top of her head. I could not see anything under the matt. "Every time I try, she growls."

I bent down for a closer look at Precious. Tangled in the hair on the top of her head, I spotted a pink ribbon. Below it, knots of fur covered a metal clip. It pulled the skin away from the skull. "Wow that must hurt." Her long hair made it impossible to see her nails. When I straightened up, our eyes met for a split second. A deep rumble started in her throat. Ed cautioned me to take her warning seriously. She bit a technician two months ago.

"OK, let me get reinforcements." I opened the door. Allie appeared with a royal blue muzzle in hand. For five minutes we tried to get the muzzle over Precious' nose. Allie held the muzzle by its long ends with her hands at the far edges. While I distracted the self-appointed queen, Allie slowly inched the muzzle toward her nose. At just the right moment, she flipped it up into position. True to form, Precious caught it in her mouth each time. During our last try, she lunged at Allie with the ferocity of a much larger animal.

I motioned for her to stop. It's humiliating when small animals outwit me. But then again, humility serves a veterinarian well. There was no choice but to knock out Precious for the procedure. Ed looked relieved as he placed her on the floor. She shook her body and walked toward the exit. In her mind, the entertainment for the day was over, and she prevailed. Little did she know what was to come.

"Not so fast, young lady." I slipped a nylon lead over her head. "You're staying with us."

After Ed left, I coaxed Precious into the treatment room. We slipped another lead over her head. Allie fastened one to the wall and held the other. Precious was stuck in the middle. While Allie distracted her, I threw a large quilt over her head and pinned her to the ground. She bit through it, narrowly missing my hand. Allie pulled up the back of the quilt and in a delightful sneak attack, injected her back leg with a sedative.

"OK, you can let her go," Allie said as she finished the injection. I jumped back but left the quilt in place as a distraction. Precious thrashed back and forth for a moment before the quilt fell off. She was mad about everything. My dignity restored, I retreated to the other, and far safer, side of the room to watch her fall asleep.

Twenty minutes later, Precious lay asleep on the treatment room table. I trimmed her nails while Allie worked on her head. The tangled hair held the clip tight against her body. Scissors were out of the question. There was no room to cut the hair without damaging her skin. The only way to free this mess was with a clipper. She would have a bald spot after we finished, and that was OK by us. Allie pushed the buzzing blade between the clip and Precious' skin. The hair gave way, revealing an inflamed patch of dermis.

For 30 minutes, Allie worked on Precious' feet. The hair between her toes twisted into thick mats. As the clipper blade became hot, she sprayed it down with lube or switched to another one. Handfuls of hair spilled off the table and covered the floor. When all the mats were gone, she trimmed up the dog's face with scissors and plucked the hair from her ears. Before Precious awoke, Allie rubbed ointment into the inflamed areas to make her more comfortable. She looked like a new dog. Sadly, her disposition was unchanged.

We must have had a sign out front that day inviting only nasty animals to enter. After Precious, Allie and I wrestled with an angry cat named Blackie. He did not want us to draw blood in an effort to check his thyroid level. Allie held Blackie on his side for a back leg draw. When the needle pierced his skin, Blackie lurched off the table with all four fangs exposed. I felt his teeth penetrate my lab coat and glide against my skin. Before I could react, Allie pulled him off my arm.

"Sorry about that, Dr. Nelson. Did he get you?" Like most medical professionals, Allie was usually unflappable, but this was too close a call. Her question conveyed genuine concern. Maintaining a vice grip on the cat, she repositioned him on the table. I pulled up my sleeve to inspect the damage. Red lines ran across the top of my hand. Thank goodness, it was only a scratch.

"We've had our share of mean animals today," I noted while cleaning my hand with antiseptic. "I'm ready for some nice ones."

After we got our draw, Allie inspected Blackie's leg and placed him in the carrier. "Well, I'm afraid we have one more to go," she replied. "You know how things seem to run in threes." She laughed and took Blackie back to his owner.

My next appointment looked simple, at least on paper. The dog needed a quick rabies vaccination before it could be placed in a permanent home by a rescue group. I entered the room, expecting a routine appointment. I should have known better.

When I opened the door, a large Rottweiler snapped to attention. His dark brown eyes stood out against his filthy coat. This dog stared at me without blinking. They were haunting, almost evil, eyes. Dominant acts by some animals are amusing; this was not. This rott truly wanted a fight with me. I kept my eyes averted in an effort to avoid provocation. Carol Donald, a petite woman with jet-black hair sat in the chair next to him. She held a chain leash with both hands.

"This is Lucifer." Naturally, I thought to myself. Carol clenched her fists around his chain leash. She explained that a neighbor called her rescue group out of concern for the dog. His owners got him as a pup and then decided he was too messy to live indoors. They chained him to a tree in the backyard without anything ... no food, water or doghouse. If it weren't for the neighbor's care, the dog would be dead.

Something about the way this dog looked at me made me wary

right from the start. Carol thought he was neglected but not abused. She said he was great with her. I decided to withhold judgment about both his attitude and her ability to restrain this dog. Lucifer weighed 110 pounds. Carol appeared to be high 90s at best. I handed her a nylon muzzle.

"Suit yourself," she replied. She placed it over the dog's mouth and fastened the strap behind his ears. As I walked around the exam room table, Lucifer and I made eye contact. We stared for about five seconds, and then he lunged at me. The chain kept him from connecting with my leg. Carol eventually pulled his head toward her lap.

"Sorry about that, Dr. Nelson," she replied in a confident voice. "I've got him now."

I crept behind him and placed my hand on his back. Lucifer's body tensed like a coiled spring. Under the thick coat, his muscles rippled. I listened to his heart, keeping my head as far away as possible. Next, I palpated his abdomen. A large scrotum hung between his back legs. Of course, his owners never had him neutered. I retreated to the other side of the table. From this safe vantage point, I noted the chain on his neck cut into his skin. His owners must have put it on him as a puppy and never bothered to expand it as he grew. Now it was embedded. The heartless treatment of his past gave me pause.

"OK, then let's give him the shot." I picked up the syringe filled with pink rabies vaccine. Carol held him like she did for the exam. I took the cap off the needle, crept around the table again and grabbed his back leg. He growled, but remained still until I stuck him with the needle. The prick provoked him. He swung his body into the wall and lunged at me. I jumped back behind the table, trembling just a bit.

"We need more help." I capped the needle and placed it on the table.

"Naw, I got him now, Doc." Carol wrapped her arms around the dog's head. "Give it another go."

"I would feel better with another set of hands and a better muzzle," I insisted. Few medals for valor are awarded in veterinary medicine. I called for Allie to bring the thick leather muzzle, the type used on police dogs. It covers the entire mouth while the nylon one lets the dog's nose stick out. Some dogs can actually bite through the narrow opening. It's more of a pinch than a bite, but it hurts.

Carol placed the leather muzzle over the nylon one and cinched down the straps. Allie put another leash around Lucifer's neck. With both women holding him in opposite directions, he was stuck in the middle where he couldn't bite either.

With everything in place, I cautiously touched his rear end. He sat down but could not spin toward me with the two leashes in place. He nervously worked to eye me. I uncapped the needle and stuck it through his skin. Lucifer let out a horrific cry and sprang into the air, pulling Carol out of her seat. He opened his mouth with such force that the rivets in the leather muzzle popped out onto the floor and hung from his neck, useless. He tore the nylon muzzle off his face with both front feet.

I retreated behind the table as Lucifer scanned the room. When his eyes settled on me, an evil expression enveloped his face. He hurled his body through the air, dragging Allie and Carol behind him. I raised my right arm in defense and braced for impact. My hand connected with his neck before his teeth reached my throat. I stiff-armed him to the side like a running back sprinting for the finish line. Lucifer turned his head and nipped my upper arm before he locked his jaws around my forearm. Searing pain rocketed through me. My arm was on fire as he crushed it between his teeth. Seconds later, my pinkie and ring fingers went numb.

Without speaking, Allie sprang to action. She pulled on the leash with all of her might. The slip lead tightened down around his neck, cutting off his air supply. When he finally gasped for air, I pulled my arm out of his mouth. I felt the skin on my arm tear away from the muscles beneath it. Pain sent me crashing backward into the wall. I struggled to stay on my feet. If I went down ...I might not get up.

"Allie, watch out," I screamed as Lucifer turned his attention to her. She slipped through the door into the lobby and slammed it on the leash, trapping the crazed dog on the other side. Lucifer spun in circles to free himself. He looked possessed. If ever a dog had the perfect name, it was this dog. Allie secured the leash to the handle. I ran out of the room, my arm limp at my side. Bright red stains appeared on the sleeve of my lab coat and kept growing as I staggered to the sink.

"Kris, are you OK?" Allie yelled from the lobby.

"I'm fine," I lied. "But check on Carol."

I teased the coat off my right arm and dropped it to the floor. Blood ran down my arm in spurts. I shoved it under the faucet without looking at the wounds. The cool water stung as it met raw tissue. My arm throbbed in unison with the beats of my heart.

"Carol is fine," Allie reported. "She's calling the rescue group to see what they want to do." She stood next to me. "How bad did he get you?"

I pulled my arm out of the sink and blotted the wounds with a paper towel. Punctures covered the area between my shoulder and wrist. He nipped me more than I realized. Blood oozed from each opening. The worst damage occurred when Lucifer locked onto my forearm – his canine teeth created two large holes in the skin. The smaller of the two was an inch in length; the big one exceeded two inches. Strands of muscle – my muscle – hung over the edges like fringe on a pillow. White bone glistened at the bottom of each hole.

At the sight of exposed bone, blood rushed from my head to my toes. My heart pounded. Surroundings faded away, and I crumpled over the sink. Allie grabbed my left arm. The room spun. I felt my body slide down the cabinets and onto the floor.

A distant voice told me to put my head between my knees. I pulled my legs toward my abdomen and leaned forward. The room kept spinning. For a moment, the pain disappeared. I felt like I was watching myself from afar. "Take deep breaths," the voice ordered. I closed my eyes and hugged my legs. "Inhale, hold it ... exhale." I tried to follow the commands. Slowly, the sense of panic left my body. I realized that I was sitting on the floor but had no idea how I got there.

"Wow," I said when I finally opened my eyes.

"Yeah, I thought you were going down for sure." Allie smiled. "You looked like those hunters who tell us all the gory details of killing an animal and then faint when they see stitches on their own dog." She let go of my arm, the one without visible bone. "I've never seen you so white."

"I felt shaky but OK until I saw the damage," I said. "Allie, it's different when it's your own body."

"Well, don't look again." Allie placed a folding chair next to me. I rested my injured arm on it. With the return of reason, I kept it higher than my heart. Allie retrieved two ice packs from the freezer, wrapped them in a towel and placed the compress on my arm. I wrapped an extra towel around my shoulders. The ice packs and ordeal made me shiver. Allie handed me a can of Sprite with orders to drink all of it. The soda made me colder still.

Our normally boisterous birds sat quietly in their cages with their eyes fixed on me, sensing that something was wrong. Bongo called out to me with the only phrase she knew, "hello, how are youuuuuuuuu?" She always drug out the word "you," which mimicked me pretty well.

"Not so good, Bongo bird," I answered.

Genny poked her head out of the office doorway. She was not used to seeing me on the ground. She sniffed my lab coat until she reached the stains. The scent of blood and mangled tissue made her raise her lips and expose her teeth. She used her front feet to roll the lab coat into a ball, with the soiled area buried in the middle, and pushed it under the counter. With that mess cleaned up, she hopped over to me and rubbed my leg. True to one of her nicknames, she was nothing if not a helper cat.

Minnesota requires 10 days of observation at an approved facility for a non-vaccinated dog who bites a human. I did not believe that punishment fit the crime. Out of concern for my well-being and because of Lucifer's remarkable strength and proven aggression, I recommended euthanasia and examination of his brain for rabies. Unfortunately, the rescue group did not agree. They thought they could rehabilitate the dog and find it a home. They wanted to "evaluate" Lucifer for themselves.

Lucifer was a loaded gun waiting to explode. It was not a matter of if, but when, he would attack again. Carol ignored my pleas and took the dog back to the rescue center. Her response left me dumbfounded.

After 15 minutes of ice, my whole arm felt numb. Before I left for the hospital, I had to flush the wounds. It is fundamental medicine. I thought of my mentor, a colorful but remarkably skilled veterinary surgeon named Lance Magnuson. Every time we worked on infected wounds, he relished imparting the maxim "the solution to pollution is dilution." Years later, I still heard his words rattle around my head every time I treated a wound. Now my arm needed a thorough cleaning. I winced at the pain to come.

As I leaned over the sink, Allie thrust the end of the drip set into the wound on top of my arm. She opened the valve wide on the bag of fluids mixed with iodine. The yellow fluid rushed into the wound. Sharp waves of pain radiated up my arm. I gritted my teeth and clenched the counter. My knuckles turned white. My body trembled.

"Are you OK?" Allie asked. I nodded without looking up. Flushing out the wound was critical to a successful outcome. I simply had to bear the pain. Bite wounds are like icebergs – the real danger hides below the surface. The mechanical action of a bite rips and destroys the tissue below. Lucifer tore my skin away from the underlying muscle and bone and crushed the muscle. The yellow fluid poured into the wound and pocketed below the skin. The pain was excruciating. With new understanding, I felt pity for my patients that have endured this procedure.

Finally, the bag emptied. Allie wrapped my arm with cast padding. Next she applied a layer of gauze followed by a product called vet wrap. She chose a bright color so I would get lots of sympathy. She held my jacket as I slid my left arm in and then hung the right side over my shoulder.

"I'd feel better if you'd let me drive you to the hospital," Allie said with emphasis.

"You need to stay here and take care of the clients." I winked at her. "I'm fine ... now that I can't see it anymore." Allie was undeterred. She studied my face intently. "But if you wouldn't mind, call Steve and let him know what happened. Try to low-key this. I know he's going to be very worried."

An hour later, I sat on a bed surrounded by plain beige curtains in Fairview's emergency room. X-rays of my arm revealed significant soft tissue swelling. With gratitude, I saw no damage to the bones and no foreign bodies. I was lucky that Lucifer did not leave any of his teeth embedded in my arm.

The ER doc had them flush my wounds again. It has always seemed that veterinarians get superior training to our human counterparts in bacteriology and the like. This flush was much less invasive, and its therapeutic efficacy questionable. The nurse held the end of the drip set over the wound and let the fluid drip onto it. When I encouraged her to place the end inside the puncture hole, she refused. She said this was how they always did it, and her decisive gestures told me that arguing was pointless. It was obvious this nurse never scrubbed with Lance.

When she left the room, I replaced the ice pack over my arm and listened to the noises around me. It sounded just like my veterinary hospital, minus barking. The familiar din comforted me. I tried to listen to the conversations and figure out the emergencies to keep my mind off my own injury. Suddenly, the curtain of my partition slid back on the metal rod. In walked Steve dressed in a suit with a green tie hanging loosely from his neck.

He put his arms around me and held me close. Tears streamed

down my face. As soon as I saw him, I could no longer control my emotions. He caressed my hair, kissed my forehead and waited for the tears to subside.

"I'm fine Sweets." I removed the ice pack from my arm and wiped my face with a tissue. "I'm just a little emotional right now."

"Understandably so," he responded, staring straight into my eyes. "How did this happen?"

Before I could answer, the emergency doc returned with a prescription for antibiotics. He chose Augmentin, the human version of my favorite antibiotic for bite wounds. He warned me to take it easy for a few days. He hoped the numbness in my pinkie and ring fingers would go away when the swelling decreased, but reminded me there were no guarantees. Lucifer might have permanently damaged the nerves to those fingers. One of my worries was my future as a surgeon. Steve now understood what hung in the balance.

"Nerve damage?" he asked as the doctor left the room.

"We'll talk on the way home," I said.

CHAPTER 10

Lucifer

T he next morning I awoke with a grotesquely large arm. Sizeable bruises covered my skin. Blood oozed from the two deepest puncture wounds, soaking the bandage. Overnight, the swelling spread from my forearm down to my fingers. I had been bitten in the past – an occupational hazard – but nothing like this. My pinkie and ring fingers had no sensation. I was scared. Just months into owning a clinic, my career might be over.

All night long, images of Lucifer haunted me. His brown eyes pierced the night like an evil spirit. I felt his gaze on me. I turned, and there he was with the worthless muzzles jangling around his neck. A second later, he transformed into a being from another world as he flew at me. I woke up kicking the covers. It was an awful night.

Loaded with Advil and antibiotics, I worked an abbreviated shift the next day. In between appointments, I sat on the floor with my arm propped up on the folding chair under an ice pack. Keeping it elevated reduced the pain by improving the circulation. Genny kept me company, playing with my leather shoelaces. Allie cancelled the week's surgical procedures. By the end of the day, the swelling was even worse. Throbbing constantly, my arm looked like it belonged to a tennis player twice my size. Despite the pain, twice a day I flushed the two puncture wounds to prevent infection. The sight of my arm prompted worry, but no longer made me faint. So far, there were no signs of overt infection although I had to assume the worst. Just like people, dogs carry bacteria in their mouths. Who knew how many microbes Lucifer injected into my arm during the attack?

The rescue group evaluated Lucifer for potential adoption and decided against it. They came to the conclusion that he was an aggressive alpha male. They felt a very large, dominant man who could put him in his place was the only kind of person who could live safely with him. He could not be trusted with women, children or other animals. Ideally, they wanted a man who lived in the countryside without any other pets or visitors. Because finding this kind of a situation was unlikely, the group relented and requested euthanasia for Lucifer.

Five days later, they brought him in wearing two heavy-duty muzzles. I slipped the noose of a rabies pole around his neck and tightened it down. With some feeling back in my right hand, I pinned him against the doorjamb. Carol held the door partially closed to protect Allie as she injected Lucifer's back leg. He assumed a defiant stance and growled at me. Saliva dripped from his lips onto the floor. Hatred filled his eyes. They seemed to glow from his head.

When the sedative took effect, Lucifer slumped onto the floor. Carol knelt over him and wept. Although she knew that euthanasia was the only viable option, she felt guilty for not being able to save Lucifer. She looked so small and frail next to the massive dog. I was thankful he never went after her. His bite would have snapped her arm like a dry twig. She left before the final injection.

Allie and I worked quickly to finish the procedure. I shaved his front leg to expose the skin. Allie placed both hands around his elbow and held off the vein. I injected the pink euthanasia fluid in one smooth motion. Lucifer took one last deep breath; then his heart stopped. He lay on the floor with his eyes open, still staring at me, piercing my soul. I shuddered. Lucifer was defiant, even in death.

Without saying a word, we slid a thick plastic body bag under his rear end. I listened to his heart with the stethoscope. I wanted to make sure he was really gone. At my word, Allie removed the muzzles and pulled the bag up over his head. She gathered the ends and twisted them together in her hands. Once the bag was closed, she applied tape with a long tag. With a thick marker she wrote "Lucifer" followed by "Rabies Suspect." I helped her place him in the large cooler.

Later that evening, Steve and I drove north from Burnsville with Lucifer's body in the trunk. We dropped it off at the University of Minnesota, College of Veterinary Medicine Diagnostic Lab (D-Lab). A veterinary student wearing dark brown coveralls (my class color was navy blue) met us at the door. The D-Lab would remove Lucifer's brain and send it to the state public health lab for further testing. After reviewing the paperwork, the student placed Lucifer in the walk-in cooler. She was blissfully unaware of the danger this dog once presented and the anxiety he wrought. To her, it was just another specimen headed to the cooler.

"You should have the results in about 10 days." She handed me a receipt. "Thanks for bringing him in."

Steve and I got back into our car without exchanging words. He watched me wiggle my fingers and touch the wounds on my arm. "Krissy, I have a special treat for you," he said.

"What kind of treat?" I asked.

"You'll just have to wait and see," was his answer.

Instead of driving south from the D-Lab back to Burnsville, he drove east through the Minnesota State Fair Grounds toward Como Park. The Veterinary College is adjacent to the fair grounds, which was always problematic when we needed to park during the fair.

For two weeks each year, the site buzzed with activity as Minnesotans celebrated all manner of food on a stick. Now the grounds were desolate; not even a stray cat was visible. Steve slowed the car to five miles below the speed limit just to be safe because the police often set up traps on the main street.

We crept over the enormous speed bumps and through the main gate. On the other side of the gate, we spotted a squad car parked along Snelling Road. Some things never change. Steve and I smiled at each other as we turned onto the busy street.

We used to take long walks around Como Park when we were dating. One glorious summer night, we found a leather wallet along the walking path. When Steve picked it up, the wallet flew out of his hand. Two teenage boys, one with a string wrapped around his hand, grabbed their bellies as they howled with delight from behind a bush. The young rascals had pulled a fast one on us. Como Park is a tranquil oasis in the City of St. Paul. Hand-in-hand, we – like many couples – loved to walk the trails around the lake.

On this night, at the corner of Lexington and Larpenteur, Steve turned left instead of right toward the park. Moments later, a familiar strip mall came into view. We were going to Ol' Mexico, one of our favorite date spots. Over chips and salsa we reminisced about some of the adventures we had shared, including our first date.

Steve and I met at a veterinary hospital. I was there to observe surgeon Lance Magnuson at the invitation of my friend and veterinary classmate, Katie. Years before, Steve started working for Lance between semesters in college. I chatted with Steve and tried not to stammer as he prepared an animal for surgery.

Steve was tall, dark and handsome. His tangible compassion for animals sealed the deal. I left the clinic in love. Unfortunately, on the ride home, Katie told me that Steve had a girlfriend. My heart sank.

Whether debriefing after a test in vet school or in matters of love, Katie was confident in her position. But she was not always correct. Steve did not have a girlfriend! In fact, about five months later, we reconnected and he wondered if I would like to carpool to work. Girls do not always get a second chance, so I did everything in my power to attract his attention. Each day, I stood for a long time at the mirror curling my hair and putting on makeup. The fact that I would cover it up with a surgical cap and mask did not matter. The more I got to know Steve, the more I liked him. Daydreams filled my thoughts ... if and when would he ask me out?

I have always been driven and worked hard for what I wanted. Three weeks after we started carpooling, I decided to see if I could speed things along. I called Steve on a Saturday afternoon to tell him I could not carpool the next day. After a few minutes of idle chatter, he asked me what I was doing for the evening. Here was my chance. I took a deep breath. "Nothing," I replied, my heart racing. "I just moved into a new apartment, so I'll probably work on the curtains and watch TV."

"You shouldn't stay home on a Saturday night," he responded. "You should go out and have fun." I jumped off the sofa with delight. My plan worked!

"Well, I would if I had someone to go with." I clung to the phone hoping beyond hope he would ask me out.

"Ah," he paused. I crossed my fingers and toes. "Well, I need to go, Kris. I'll see you tomorrow." He sounded nervous and hung up. That was it. No invitation. I felt my heart sink again. For the next 24 hours I dissected our conversation. Everything seemed to be going perfectly. What went wrong? Perhaps I had been too aggressive and scared him off. Perhaps I sounded too desperate. I worried I would never get a chance to date him. Thank goodness, Steve had other ideas.

After our shift ended on Sunday, Steve asked me if I'd like to listen to some jazz music at the Music Festival on Cedar Avenue. I agreed, of course, thrilled beyond words that he asked me out. Unfortunately, all we could find at the festival were country-western bands catering to bikers. Our jeans and polo shirts stuck out among the leather and studs. Neither one of us felt particularly safe, so we decided on an alternate plan.

"How about dinner?" Steve suggested since the music was a bust. "I know a great place on the river by St. Anthony Falls."

Close to the lock and dam, this had never been a great neighborhood. We drove down a dark abandoned street that was eerily quiet. From the glow of a harvest moon, we could just make out the boarded-up windows of this once-thriving hotspot. Some first date. With two strikes against him, Steve panicked. The only way to salvage this date was to spend some serious money on dinner.

At 8:45 p.m., we walked into a French café named Yvette's. The manager escorted us to a romantic table on the patio. We sat next to the sidewalk with a beautiful view of the river and city skyline. The falls rumbled in the background.

Halfway through the meal, two homeless men approached our table from the street. They smelled rancid. They stopped on the other side of the railing that separated the tables from the street. At first, they just looked at us.

"Get out," the taller one ordered, slurring his words. The smell of alcohol clung to his breath.

"Excuse me?" Steve answered.

"I told you to get out. We live here, and you don't. So ..." He stopped talking and stared at me. He raised his hand and pointed at my face. I leaned back in my chair, away from this strange man. I grew up in the country, on a hobby farm with lots of animals. Homeless people from the city were not part of any experience I could draw on for insight. I was unsure how to respond or what to do. "Hey," he drawled on before I could react, "she's pretty."

"I know," Steve replied. "That's why I asked her out." My heart jumped for joy, but I was still scared and uncertain. "As soon as we finish dinner, we will leave. I'm sorry that we came into your home uninvited," Steve continued, trying to placate them. The men looked at each other but did not leave. To my horror, they moved even closer to me.

"OK, move it along," a voice commanded from across the street. Two police officers approached the pair and escorted them away. After they were gone, Steve apologized for the evening. I could see the agony on his face for everything that had gone wrong. He felt horrible about the evening. I, on the other hand, liked how it was progressing.

"I just wanted to spend time with you," I answered and smiled at him so my dimples showed. "I really didn't care what we did." Steve reached across the table and took my hand in his. My whole body exploded with a rush. It was the perfect moment and perfect ending to a memorable first date.

Now, enjoying dinner at Ol' Mexico, Steve kept me thinking about the fun and silly things we did when we were dating. By the time we left the restaurant, I forgot all about Lucifer and the ordeal of euthanizing him. For the first time since the attack, I slept peacefully through the night.

CHAPTER 11

Cosmo Saves Us

With only a day to go before the big Wisconsin hunt, Bridget's paw was still a problem. I listed her as questionable for the trip. Since her last visit, I had left the wound open under a light protective wrap. Joe and Sally tended to her paw faithfully and called me with updates. Today was crunch time. The hunting party departed tomorrow morning.

The entire Smith family escorted Bridget into the hospital. She wore a freezer bag over her bandage to protect it from the slushy conditions. The night before, a light blanket of snow had fallen. The morning sun melted the beautiful white flakes into a gray slush that coated everything.

Some hunting dogs spend their lives in a kennel, never venturing indoors. Their owners consider them tools for the hunt, nothing more. They are a commodity – valuable ones – but still just that. I could spot these kennel dogs every time because they basked in the attention they received at the clinic. We showered them with hugs, reassuring pats and biscuits. Some of the owners told us to knock it off. They believed that spoiling the dog with attention would ruin their desire to hunt. To their mind, a dog could not be a pet and also perform well in the field. As one trainer with a chrome whistle hanging around his neck told me, "Once they sleep on the couch, they're ruined forever."

Bridget Smith threw this theory right out the window. She lived indoors with her human family on a lovely wooded lot. As the first "baby" of the family, she enjoyed life to the fullest. She went everywhere with Joe and Sally. At Christmas, a stocking hung above the fireplace with her name on it. She even got to sleep on the bed when Joe was away on business.

But when Bridget hit the field, she was all business. She pointed, flushed and retrieved birds with gusto. Her desire to please was remarkable. She let nothing stand between her and the bird. I wished that trainer with the chrome whistle could see her in action. The strong bond Bridget shared with her family made her an unbelievable hunting dog. She would do anything to please them. Now this endearing trait concerned me. I knew she would hunt through the pain of her foot no matter what. I would have to be super cautious with her.

Bridget lay on her side with her head in Joe's lap as I removed the bandage. The surface of the central pad had improved greatly. It was thicker and firm to the touch. The actual wound was now about half as long as the original gash.

"So far, so good," I announced after inspecting the surface of her paw. Joe patted her head again. All of the sensation had returned to my right hand after the incident with Lucifer, and I no longer took the use of fingers for granted. With my thumb and index finger I gently spread open the edges of the wound. The original hole extended deep into the tissue, almost slicing the pad in half. To my relief, pink healthy granulation tissue now filled the void.

"Much better," I stated, still examining her paw. "The wound had healed from the inside out like I'd hoped. It's about 75 percent closed." I put down her paw. "Just the surface remains to heal."

"Does that mean she can go?" Joe asked.

"I think so," I answered. He beamed from ear to ear. I warned Joe and Sally that they'd have to take special precautions to protect the foot. Bridget would need to wear a protective bootie with a non-skid sole on her foot. I wanted them to inspect her paw every two hours. If the wound deepened, she would have to retire for the day.

Sensing Joe's excitement, Bridget sat up and licked his face. The entire family hugged her. Joe and Sally always carried a first-aid kit in their pack. They would add a few dog-specific items, just in case. And they promised to bring her back to camp if the wound worsened.

"Joe, one last thing before you go," I said. The couple turned to look at me. "No more pad lacerations right before the big trip. I don't need that kind of pressure in my life." The entire Smith family laughed. They valued Bridget's health and well-being more than anything. I knew they would be hyper-vigilant with her on the trip. "Have a wonderful time."

"You're supposed to wish us a successful hunt," Sally responded.

"Sorry, but I can't do that. I always cheer for the animals." I smiled. "No offense, but I hope you come home birdless." The family laughed again.

When I was young, maybe 5 or 6, my Dad took me duck hunting. I set up a hospital in the bow of the boat with blankets, bits of bread and water. When a dog brought a bird in, I dressed its wounds and tried to save it. I wanted to save them all. I still do.

The other men in the group gave my Dad a hard time about my "hospital." They weren't too excited about having a little girl along in the first place. Prior to the "hospital," I tried scaring away the ducks with non-stop chatter. When Dad ended that rebellion, I quietly gathered the medical tools in the bow, hoping to save any bird that was shot. For my Dad and his friends, the "hospital" was the last straw. I never received another invitation to hunt.

Bridget pranced out of the building wearing a new bandage and plastic bag. The mail lady watched her go as she entered the building. Ann Delaney loved coming into our office and seeing all the animals. When Romeo the bird was in the lobby, she always stayed an extra minute to talk to him. He responded with chirps and squeaks.

"What's wrong with that dog?" she asked as she placed a stack of letters on the counter.

"She lacerated the big middle pad on her foot," I replied as I picked up the stack of mail.

"This Norfolk pine looks sick." She pointed to the plant. "You should really move it away from the window to a more protected area. They like tropical conditions." She readjusted the leather strap from the mailbag as her glasses fogged in the clinic's warm air.

"I did not know that," I said. "We'll move it right away."

Ann nodded and headed out the door.

An official-looking letter with the return address of Minnesota State Public Health Laboratory lay on the top of the stack. I ripped open the envelope and pulled out the letter. The results of the fluorescent antibody test for Lucifer were negative. He did not have rabies! Finally, some good news involving that wretched dog.

Buoyed by the news, I opened another official-looking envelope from a legal firm. "Dear Dr. Nelson," the letter began. "On behalf of my client, I am immediately ordering you to cease and desist using the name Minnesota Veterinary Center." I continued to read in disbelief. Another clinic with a similar name threatened to sue me if I did not change the name of my hospital.

Running through my mind was a tally of the precious money I spent on a sign, letterhead, business cards and the like. After selecting the name "Minnesota Veterinary Center," I checked with the secretary of state to make sure the name was available. When it was, I paid the fee and registered it. Why would this clinic on the opposite side of the Twin Cities do this? After all, there were other veterinary entities with "Minnesota" in their names.

I called my attorney for advice. He suggested changing the

name to avoid a legal fight. In his opinion, this choice offered the path of least resistance since the clinic was so new. I decided against it. After all the time and money I had put into the name, I didn't want to change it now. Nor could I afford to. I held my ground and asked him to respond with a stern letter.

As a young business owner, I had already had people try to take advantage of me. One company sent an unordered box of exam gloves to the clinic. Later, we received a bill for more than $200 from the company. A box of these gloves typically goes for less than $10.

In addition, sales reps descended on the clinic like vultures on roadkill. They showed up without appointments and referred to me as "honey," "missy" and "dear." When I refused to speak with them, they stormed out of the clinic upset at my ostensibly rude behavior.

My scariest incident happened with a man selling office supplies. He wore a black wool coat over a pinstripe suit with a bright red tie. He slicked his hair down with a flourish over his forehead and topped off the outfit with a gold chain on his right wrist. He placed his briefcase on the counter and pulled out an assortment of brochures even though Allie told him we weren't interested. He refused to leave until he spoke with the owner.

I marched into the lobby, steaming. "My name is Dr. Nelson," I announced. "I am the owner of this clinic, and I am not interested in anything you have to sell. Please leave now." The man did not budge.

"Missy, you're only saying that because you don't know what I have to offer," he countered.

"Leave now and never come back," I said icily. "I will not buy anything from you."

"Honey, I love a challenge." He smiled. "I'm not leaving until you buy your office supplies from me." He looked at me with an almost sinister gaze.

"Fine, I'll have the police escort you out then." I turned and headed out of the lobby into the pharmacy area. Allie closed the door behind me. As I picked up the receiver, we heard a loud creak. The salesman opened the door!

"Let Cosmo out," I whispered to Allie. She hurried off. "I told you to leave," I yelled, facing him with the receiver in my hand. "Take one more step, and I'm calling the police."

"Sweetie," he smiled at me. "There is no need to do that." He froze in the doorway with his hand on the doorknob. "Now let me show you how my products will help your business."

Inside the first run, Cosmo, a pit bull snoozed on a blanket. His massive muscles bulged beneath his tawny brown coat. The large dog had lacerated his right hock a month before. It became infected and was not healing. Today his owner had dropped him off for surgical debridement of the wound. Allie opened the gate to his run.

"Come, Cosmo." She patted her hip. He sprang to his feet and bounded over the kennel threshold. Allie ran to the pharmacy with Cosmo tight on her heels. The youngster loved to play. He loped behind her with a silly grin. His tongue hung out the side of his mouth and dripped saliva on the floor.

When they reached the pharmacy, Cosmo skidded to a halt in the middle of the room. The smile on his face vanished. He stared at the salesman without blinking. The hair on his back stood up. I walked over to his side and put my hand on him.

"Go now, or I'll release the dog," I told the salesman. As if on cue, Cosmo pulled his lips back to display gleaming white teeth. A low growl rumbled from his throat. Animals are amazing. This happy-go-lucky pup transformed into a guard dog at the critical moment.

The man retreated behind the door and slammed it shut. We stood frozen in place until the doorbell dinged. I threw my arms around Cosmo's neck and hugged him. He turned his head and licked the side of my face with his massive tongue. Allie scratched his back with both hands. He arched his back and closed his eyes from the attention.

"I'm sure glad he was here." Allie continued to scratch his back. "Did you see the look on that guy's face? You scared him witless, Cosmo."

"Serves him right," I said. I pushed a stray strand of hair behind my ear. "Why do some men try to take advantage of us? No means no."

"Especially when the woman saying it has a pit bull waiting in back," Allie added. We smiled and looked at Cosmo. He returned the gaze for a few seconds with his ears perked forward, then relaxed into a big doggy grin. The salesman never returned.

CHAPTER 12

Blake's Christmas Puppy

With Christmas right around the corner, our phone rang off the hook. People wanted last-minute appointments. Some animals needed vaccinations before the boarding kennel would take them. Others needed health certificates for travel out of state. But the majority of people scheduled examinations for pets that were Christmas presents. My next appointment was a new puppy exam – something I thoroughly enjoy.

Blake Thomas, a 4th-grader, wanted a puppy more than anything in the world. He checked out books from the elementary school library to learn how to train a puppy. Every week, he saved a portion of his allowance for toys, a collar and a matching leash. Blake's mother, Jennifer, decided he was finally old enough to care for a pet. This year, he would get a puppy for Christmas. The single mother and son purchased a Bernese mountain dog, Captain, from a local breeder. He looked like a black teddy bear with rust and white highlights.

Captain wiggled back and forth on the exam table as I entered the room. Every time I looked into his eyes, his tongue popped out of his mouth to lick me. The faint smell of puppy breath filled the room. Jennifer handed me his papers. The breeder had dewormed Captain and given him the first set of vaccinations. All he needed today was a physical examination.

"Would you like to help me?" I looked at Blake and waited for his response. He jumped off the chair and knocked his backpack to the ground. "I want you to hold Captain's head so I can examine his eyes and ears." The boy stood on his tiptoes and put his hands of both sides of Captain's face. I looked down the pup's ears and into his beautiful brown eyes. Next, I opened his mouth with both hands. Small sparkling baby teeth lined the jaws. The pup tried to chew on my fingers.

"No, you don't, young man," I admonished. "Those deciduous teeth are too sharp for that."

"You're right about that, Dr. Nelson," Jennifer agreed. "Blake, honey, show Dr. Nelson your arms." He pulled back the sleeves of his winter jacket. Long red scratches covered his hands and forearms.

"Oh my, it looks like Captain thinks you're a chew toy. You shouldn't let him chew on you like that," I said. Blake let his sleeves slide down into place and looked at the floor.

"I've told Blake over and over again not to play rough like that, but he ignores me," Jennifer said. "Any suggestions?"

"Rub a little lemon juice on Blake's hands and arms," I responded quietly. "Most dogs hate the bitter taste of lemon." Jennifer nodded and ran her hand down Captain's back. I listened to the puppy's heart with the stethoscope that always hung around my neck. When finished, I decided to do something special for Blake.

When I was 4 years old, our family veterinarian noticed me peering over the table as he examined our pet. Babbette, our miniature black poodle, sat on the table with her eyes focused on the door to the waiting room. Babbette hated her annual trip to the vet's office. Dr. Anderson spoke to her in soothing tones as he looked in her eyes and ears. She panted and eyed him nervously. When he pulled a stethoscope out of the drawer in the table, Babbie ran to the end of the table. He plucked her from the air just before she hit the ground.

"She certainly is a feisty dog," he commented, returning her to the table. His salt-and-pepper hair reminded me of a schnauzer I saw in his waiting room.

"And she bites sometimes, too," I added.

"That's only when you bother her, Krissy," my mom added. "When she goes behind the couch, she wants to be left alone." Dr. Anderson looked at my mom and smiled. As the father of three boys, he knew all about kids. Even though he was perfectly capable of handling Babbie by himself, Dr. Anderson asked me to hold her.

I stood on my tiptoes and placed my hands around the poodle's neck. She panted at an even faster rate than before. When he finished with Babbie's vaccinations, he invited my family to the back of the clinic to see the animals. I poked my finger through the cage doors and petted the dogs and cats inside. One handsome orange tabby licked my finger.

"You have a way with animals, young lady," Dr. Anderson stated. He looked so impressive in his white lab coat. "Thanks for helping me with your dog." I beamed and looked at the floor.

"Krissy, thank Dr. Anderson for giving us a tour." My mom was diligent about manners.

"Thank you," I mumbled, still looking at the floor. When I saw him leave the room, I turned to my mother and pulled on her purse. "Mom, when I grow up, I'm going to be a veterinarian like Dr. Anderson."

"That's nice, dear," she responded while rummaging for the car keys.

"No, Mom, I really mean it. I'm going to be a veterinarian." She stopped and looked at me with her hand still inside the purse. "I said that's nice; now button your jacket. Babbie wants to go home." I trailed behind her through the door. I knew she didn't believe me, but that didn't dampen my spirits. On that day, in that exam room, I decided to become a vet. Now, 28 years later, a diploma from the University of Minnesota, College of Veterinary Medicine, hung on the wall in my own waiting room. The dream had come true!

I saw the same spark in Blake and wanted to encourage him as Dr. Anderson had me.

"Would you like to listen to Captain's heart?" I asked. His eyes widened. He nodded his head like a bobblehead doll. I placed the tips of the stethoscope in Blake's ears and held the bell over Captain's heart. "Captain's heart sounds like a loud lub, dub, lub dub," I instructed. "Do you hear that?" He smiled and nodded. After a minute, he removed the tips from his ears with both hands.

"That was cool!" he exclaimed.

With the stethoscope back around my neck, I finished the examination. Captain looked great. I could not find any problems. I opened a drawer and pulled out two dog biscuits. I asked Blake to promise he would take good care of this precious bundle of fur.

"Cross my heart and hope to die," Blake answered while crossing his heart with his hand.

I smiled in response and placed one biscuit on the table. The pup sniffed twice, then clamped down on the treat. Brown crumbs fell from his mouth onto the table. He vacuumed those up then looked at me for more. "You like treats, don't you, hot stuff?" I said. Captain jumped up and grabbed the black tubing of the stethoscope. I quickly freed it from his jaws. Small indentations from his baby teeth covered the black tubing, but none penetrated to the interior. "No more treats for you if you grab my stethoscope. That is not a puppy toy."

A loud crash reverberated from the waiting room, followed by footsteps. Five seconds later, we heard Allie yell the word, "No!"

"What was that?" Jennifer asked.

"Sounds like Scruffy got into trouble again." I laughed. "He's a stray cat that needs a home." I looked at Jennifer. "Would you like to adopt him? Perhaps Captain needs a brother?"

"Yeah, Mom, Captain needs a brother," Blake repeated. He held his mother's hand and looked into her face with pleading eyes.

"Oh no, one puppy is more than enough right now. Between working full time and taking care of you, I don't have time to do anything else," she replied. She promised to mention Scruffy if she ran into anyone who wanted a cat.

Since his arrival at the clinic, the emaciated kitten had doubled his weight. Scruffy had morphed into a handsome boy with a mischievous personality. He loved to knock things off the counter, including plastic tops from the syringe cases. Once they landed on the ground, he batted them through the clinic like hockey pucks. We found them under chairs, in the bathroom and even behind the dryer. Allie hung a syringe case with medical tape from the front of his cage. Scruffy spent hours on his back, pawing the toy. He loved hearing it clink against the bars.

After his first bath, Scruffy worked hard to keep himself clean. He spent hours each day grooming his coat until the white sparkled. He kept each hair in place, using his paws to reach the tough areas. His attention to cleanliness bordered on fanaticism. He loved being clean!

Scruffy's confidence grew with his stature. He prowled the clinic like a king surveying his territory. His life was perfect ... well almost perfect. If only Genny would play with him. He wanted to wrestle with her in the worst way, but Genny would have nothing to do with him. The precocious teenager did not want to share her territory with any other cat. She considered herself superior to all, including me. She despised Scruffy for not acknowledging her preeminent position. In her mind, he was lower than dirt. Not just any dirt, mind you, but the filthy kind found on Minnesota roads once the snow melts.

With patience, most cats adjust to living with others. They work out boundaries of behavior and space acceptable to everyone. Besides being an orphan with a limited understanding of feline etiquette, Genny's physical condition challenged her ability to deal with Scruffy. She limped around the clinic on her left back leg, carrying her stump in the air. Often, she lay on her side, giving her good leg a rest. With only three legs, she was no match for the young and fully mobile Scruffy. The situation was clear. The first animal to join the family takes precedence. So with heavy hearts, Allie and I put the word out. Scruffy needed a home of his own.

The week before Christmas, Mike Kinney, a friend of Allie's, stopped by the clinic with his girlfriend Theresa Hoffman to meet Scruffy. Allie took the couple to Scruffy's cage. He found himself locked up again after knocking the appointment book off the counter. When Allie withdrew Scruffy from the cage and put him on the table, he immediately jumped onto Mike's shoulders. The cat purred and rubbed his face against the young man's beard. Mike laughed and petted him with one hand. Scruffy responded by licking his ear. Allie pulled Scruffy off and put him on the table again.

"I've never seen Scruffy do that before," she commented. "He really likes you."

Mike beamed. "Why do you call him Scruffy? He's a really handsome cat, not at all what I pictured from your description."

Allie explained that Scruffy's nickname was due to his appearance when she found him. His new owners could change it to whatever they wanted by coupling Scruffy with the new name for a while. When he caught on to the combination name, they could drop the nickname. Based on her observations of him in the clinic, she thought he was an intelligent cat. He should catch on without any problem.

Mike's girlfriend Theresa was concerned about Scruffy's health, wondering if he'd suffer any long-term problems. Allie explained that Scruffy's blood work looked great, so we thought he would be fine. He tested negative for feline leukemia, feline immunodeficiency virus and feline infectious peritonitis, the three most common infectious diseases in strays. He'd already had his first set of vaccinations and had finished his medicine to get rid of intestinal parasites. "If you adopt him, Dr. Nelson said she would give him his last set of shots and neuter him for free on one condition."

"What's that?" the couple asked in unison.

"You have to call us with updates and bring him back here for his shots." She petted the cat. "We're really going to miss him."

With his sweet personality, handsome appearance, heart-breaking story and award-winning performance, Scruffy captured Mike's heart straight away. It was a perfect match. With his girl-friend's blessing, Mike decided to adopt Scruffy on the spot.

"Can I take him with me now?" he asked, holding Scruffy in his arms.

Allie recommended later in the week, after his neuter. That would give Scruffy time to heal and Mike time to catproof his house. Mike reluctantly agreed. He kissed the cat goodbye and put him back in the cage. When Scruffy's feet hit the cage bottom, he spun around and tried to jump back into Mike's arms. Allie was too quick and managed to close the door. Foiled by a wily techni-cian, Scruffy stood on his hind legs and reached through the bars with his front paws to touch Mike's arm, meowing pitifully.

"Don't worry, pal; you won't be stuck here much longer." Mike petted him through the bars. "You'll be home for Christmas."

CHAPTER 13

Oscar the Parrot

"Thank you for fitting Chiffon in on such short notice," Jerry Cummings said. The man looked worn out, like he'd been through the wringer and barely made it back. "Her regular clinic is already closed."

"No problem," Allie answered. Reindeer decorated her scrubs. The one on her front pocket had a red sequin sewn over its nose. She studied the new client sheet Jerry had completed. The little Maltese fit in the palm of his hand. She was current on all of her shots and heartworm protection. Jerry brought her in for an examination of her rear end. The 5-month-old puppy cried when she defecated. The owner thought she needed her glands squeezed.

Jerry peeled Chiffon off his shoulder and placed her on the scale. She danced on it for a minute before settling down. Her little body tipped the scale at two-and-a half pounds.

"If it's OK with you, I'm going to put you two in the cat room. I haven't had time to clean the dog room," Allie explained. "It's actually a better exam room because of the aquarium." She opened the door and escorted the pair into the room. It had the same color scheme as the dog room – sky blue on the bottom and white upper walls. The only difference was the border – kittens with balls of yarn instead of hunting dogs and decoys. The corner of the room featured a 20-gallon aquarium. Inside, four small gold angelfish swam from side to side. I was told angel-fish don't fight unless they pair up, so I bought five for the tank. Within a week, one fish was missing. Some pet store clerks are more knowledgeable than others.

Jerry showed Chiffon the tank. The pup touched her nose to the glass, and all the fish scattered except one. The biggest swam straight toward the pup, flaring his fins and acting like a raging bull elephant. Chiffon barked twice, but the fish held its ground. This fish was fearless.

"Now, I just have a few more questions before Dr. Nelson comes in to examine your dog." Allie looked at the info sheet again. "I can't quite make out what you wrote here. Who is Chiffon's owner?"

The man nodded. "Yes, I know it's a little confusing," he said. "Chiffon belongs to my daughter." He took a deep breath. "My daughter, Julie, is very ill. She can't even leave her house anymore. I decided to get her a dog to see if that would lift her spirits. She always wanted one of these little yappers." He looked down at the white ball of fur in his arms. Chiffon looked like a fluffy snowball.

He explained that Chiffon found her new home a little over-whelming at first. The medical equipment terrified her. She barked every time a monitor beeped and ran for cover. The tall hospital bed presented another problem. Chiffon was too small to jump onto the bed. Jerry bought a carpet-covered ramp for her and placed it by the bed. Chiffon learned to run up and down the ramp for a treat. Her playful spirit was a breath of fresh air for the bedridden woman. Chiffon gave her a reason to live.

Allie took a thermometer out of the drawer. "OK, I need to take her temperature, and then I'll get Dr. Nelson." Jerry held the dog with her rear end toward Allie. She lifted the tail with one hand to insert the thermometer with the other. With every attempt, the pup squealed.

"I'm not sure if she's acting, or if something is really wrong," Allie said. "I think I'll let Dr. Nelson take her temperature."

Allie held Chiffon for the examination while Jerry relaxed in the chair. I started at her head and worked toward her tail. She looked great until I got to her hindquarters. The area on both sides of her anus swelled out from her body. I put on a pair of gloves and gently pressed on the area. It felt soft and squishy. The next thing I noticed was the small size of the dog's anus. The diameter was the size of a pen, about half as big as I expected. I inserted the tip of the thermometer through the opening. It felt tight, not elastic like a normal anus.

"Well, I'm afraid Chiffon's problem is more severe than full anal glands," I explained while removing my gloves. Allie cleaned the rear with a moist paper towel. Chiffon's anus was very small, making it difficult for her to defecate. She had to push with all her might to force the stool through the narrow opening. The pushing put extra pressure on the muscles around her anus. Eventually, they gave out, and hernias formed.

"What can you do for her?" Jerry took the dog from Allie. "It would kill my daughter if something happened to her." No pressure here, I thought. I recalled the retired woman who told me I "had to save her dog" because it was the last living connection to her husband. They picked him out together at a nearby shelter. A month later, her husband died. Lucky for me, the dog had something I could treat. I dread the day he develops something I cannot.

"I need to do a contrast study of the area to confirm my diagnosis," I explained. "If I'm right, I will refer you to a specialist for surgical correction. In the meantime, I'm going to put her on a stool softener called lactulose. It will make it easier for her to defecate."

"Can't you do the surgery, Dr. Nelson?" Jerry asked. "You are so gentle with little Chiffon, I would feel more comfortable if you did it."

I shook my head. "That is so kind, but it will be better for

Chiffon if I refer her out. Fixing those hernias and opening up her anus requires a surgeon with a lot of experience. I have assisted on enough of them to know it is something for an expert." I smiled at Jerry. "But the good news is that I believe we can make her better. So tell your daughter not to worry."

"Too late," he replied.

We made arrangements to perform the barium study the next morning, on Christmas Eve. In the meantime, he would give Chiffon the medicine and page me if she had any problems. While he paid for his visit, Jerry placed Chiffon on the lobby floor. She ran in ever-expanding circles around his feet. Genny sat above her on the counter. Normally, she would hop into the back, away from the annoying youngster, but today, she stayed put. While Allie helped Jerry, Genny crept to the Christmas tree on the counter. The miniature ornaments fascinated her. She batted at a gold bell and waited for Allie to respond. When she didn't, Genny grabbed the ornament in her teeth and high-tailed it for the back.

"Genny," Allie shouted. She looked at Jerry and shrugged. "That's the fourth ornament she's grabbed today. I can't wait until we put that tree away." Jerry smiled, happy that Chiffon couldn't jump onto counters or he'd have a similar problem.

"See you tomorrow," he responded and walked into the crisp Minnesota air.

The next day Jerry dropped off Chiffon at 9 a.m. sharp. Much to my relief, her medical condition was not as severe as I feared. When the last film hung from the X-ray viewer, I felt a lot better about Chiffon's condition. While she was out, I passed my gloved pinky finger into her anus and palpated the area. Her anus was bigger than I thought, and the hernias were smaller. I couldn't wait to tell Jerry. Although she still needed surgery, her chances for a complete cure were good. I dialed Jerry from the treatment room to share the results.

"Oh, that is good news. My daughter will be so happy," he commented. A loud scream echoed through the clinic. "What was that?" he asked, alarmed.

"That's Oscar," I replied. "He's a very unhappy Severe Macaw."

"Wow, I'm glad he doesn't live with me."

"Yes, he's a real handful," I said. Oscar squawked again. Even though he was a room away, he sounded like he was right next to me. Of all the birds I have ever worked with, he was the loudest. I quickly said goodbye to Jerry before Oscar could scream again.

The hands on Allie's Star Trek watch read 4:00 p.m. when Jerry arrived at the clinic. After he paid the bill, Allie took him in back to see the films. In the pharmacy area, she stopped to show him the clinic birds. Besides Bongo, Windsor and Romeo, I also had a border canary I adopted during my internship at the Animal Medical Center in New York City. Then, there was Oscar.

"Which one is the screamer?" he asked.

She pointed at a large green bird with a red head. "Oscar can rock the rafters when he gets going. Dr. Nelson rescued him from a garage." She looked into the bird's cage. He perched on a natural branch that ran from side to side. He constricted and dilated his pupils in response to Allie but, thank goodness, did not scream. "You be a good bird, Oscar; I'll feed you in a few minutes."

"Good bird, good bird," Bongo repeated.

"Which one said that?" Jerry asked. His eyes darted between the cages.

Allie pointed at a slightly smaller green bird with a yellow head and short tail. Bongo paced back and forth on her perch, upset that Allie was paying attention to Oscar instead of her. "Yes, Bongo is a good bird if you don't scream like Oscar." They laughed and walked back to the treatment room.

When Chiffon saw Jerry, she stood on her back legs and pawed the air with her front feet. Allie opened the cage and handed her over. The excited pup licked every part of the man's face she could reach. Her tail whipped back and forth as fast as she could wag it.

"I think she missed you," Allie said.

"Yes, it seems so." Jerry looked at Scruffy curled up in a blanket in the cage below. "Looks like you had some company in here,

Chiffon. What's wrong with that cat? He looks kind of out of it."

Allie explained that Scruffy was recovering from a neuter. She reached her finger through the bars and rubbed his forehead. He purred and closed his eyes. His new owner would pick him up on his way home from work. Allie then excused herself to feed the birds.

I motioned to Jerry to join me at the viewer. We looked at each film, one by one. I traced organs with my finger as I explained the images. Jerry listened intently with Chiffon perched on his shoulder.

Suddenly, Allie screamed from the pharmacy area. "Dr. Nelson, help!" Chiffon hid her face under Jerry's. I ran by him without excusing myself. When I reached the pharmacy area, I saw Oscar's cage door hanging open. My heart raced. I scanned the room, looking for Allie.

Inside my office, Allie stood on a folding chair. Oscar marched around the bottom of the chair with his wings out in full attack position. Every few steps he stopped and stared up at Allie with his beak open.

"What happened?" I asked, trying to stifle a laugh.

"He snuck out of the cage and climbed to the ground when I went to feed him. When I tried to put him back in, he chased me. I jumped on the chair to get away," Allie said.

I held my lips together and closed my eyes. I knew she was really upset, but this was hysterical. The bird weighed less than a pound but had treed a human! Allie looked at me and knew I was laughing. "It's not funny," she continued. "Look what he did to my shoe." She pointed to the heel of her shoe. Two deep V's marked the rubber, compliments of Oscar's upper and lower beaks.

I walked over to Oscar and stuck my hand in front of his chest. "Step up!" I ordered. Vets learn to always sound confident. Internally, anything goes, but to the outside world we are calm and in control. I was not the least bit certain this bird would obey. I had only been teaching him the command for about a week. Oscar lifted his left foot, placed it on my cupped hand and stepped up off the floor. I carried him back to the cage, still trying to suppress my laughter. Allie waited until I had completely secured the cage door before she descended from the safety of the chair. Jerry stood in the doorway with Chiffon in his arms, his mouth hanging wide open.

I explained that Oscar chose me for his mate since there were no female macaws available. As is common with birds, he considers everyone else competition for my attention. That's why he attacked Allie. Oscar, The Jealous did not want to share me with anyone else. Jerry stood motionless, apparently still in shock.

"The good news is, I found a home for him on the other side of Minneapolis. Soon Oscar will have a real girlfriend."

"Not soon enough," Allie muttered as she walked past me. "Not soon enough."

CHAPTER 14

Moe the Ferret

With the holidays complete, Minnesotans settle in for the long winter. The change in mood, like the change in sunlight, is discernable and bleak. In January, the sun sets around 5 p.m. each day and does not reappear until 7:30 the next morning. A thick layer of ice blankets the snow, crunching under your feet with each step. At night, temperatures often plunge below zero. Most days, the air warms to the teens. It's often too cold to snow!

To deal with the extreme cold, most people winterize their cars, replacing the summer oil with a lighter variety. Minnesotans store blankets, shovels and kitty litter in the trunk, just in case the car gets stuck. In the glove compartment, most drivers stash an emergency food supply. The frozen candy bars rattle around until spring. On the floor rests an ice scraper. The complimentary version has a company logo painted on the plastic face. The fancy variety sold at every gas station has a brush attached to the other end.

Some cars are equipped with an engine-block heater. You can tell by the short black cord sticking out from the grill of the car. Upscale parking lots provide outlets for each space. Truly upscale garages are enclosed, heated and have valets.

Steve and I slept under two blankets and a thick quilt. Although both of us grew up in Minnesota, we despised the cold, never acclimating to it like our friends. While they went ice fishing, skiing and snowmobiling, we stayed inside, drank hot chocolate by the fire and dreamed of Hawai'i – our honeymoon destination years before. Shoveling snow was more outdoor activity than we wanted in the bitter months.

Despite the exhaustion common among new business owners, we sometimes found it hard to sleep. The clinic was progressing, but money was tight ... very tight. Year-end and the obligatory Christmas expenses caused a good deal of anxiety. We hoped the practice would continue to grow and do so rapidly enough to keep us afloat.

"Beep, beep, beep," the pager sounded from the nightstand one bitterly cold night. I struggled to turn off the device in the dark. "Beep, beep, beep." It continued to pierce the silence. I pulled the cord on the lamp on the nightstand, almost knocking over the clock in the process. When my eyes adjusted to the light, I switched off the pager and studied the number. I did not recognize it.

"Hello," a masculine voice answered.

"Hello, this is Dr. Nelson calling. Did you call for a veterinarian?"

"Kris, I'm sorry to bother you, but Moe is really sick." Moe, I thought to myself. I couldn't place the name or the voice. I thought for a minute before the caller continued as if reading my mind. "Moe, the sable ferret that you always confuse with my albino ferrets, Curly and Larry." The cobwebs lifted and an image of the ferrets appeared in my consciousness.

"Sorry, Scott, I'm not awake yet. What's going on with Moe?"

Scott told me that the ferret was salivating and pawing at his mouth. He stopped eating two days ago after chewing up a rubber dinosaur. He started vomiting this morning.

"Scott, why did you wait so long to call? You know better than that."

"I know, but I'm short on cash. I was hoping it would pass on its own." He paused for a minute. "Do you think he can wait until the morning?"

"Well, that depends," I answered. "Pull up the skin on his back and let it go. Does it snap right back into place?" I waited for Scott's response.

"Its' staying pulled up," he finally replied.

Bummer, I thought.

I then had him check Moe's mouth and gums. He reported that Moe's gums were light pink in color. When he pressed on the gum, it took about two seconds for the light pink color to return. Finally I inquired about his demeanor. I wanted to know if he was his normal busy self or was just lying there. Scott reluctantly reported that Moe was depressed. This mischievous little ferret let him open his mouth without even trying to get away. Scott agreed to meet me at the clinic as quickly as possible.

I hung up the phone and rubbed my eyes. The digital clock read1:30 a.m. When I worked at the emergency clinic, we always got a flurry of activity after the bars closed. I wished the legislature would establish an earlier last call law. The animals wouldn't have to suffer as long, and the veterinarians would get more sleep.

"Steve." I put my hand on his shoulder. "You've got to get up. We need to go to the clinic." I looked at him and waited a minute for a response. He continued to sleep as only he could. I pulled the covers from his shoulders. He finally opened his eyes. "I think a ferret needs surgery. It sounds pretty bad."

"OK, I'll be there in a minute," he mumbled, pulling the quilt over his shoulders again. "You can have the bathroom first."

"Nice try, Sweets." I walked around the bed to his side, shivering against the cold. I pulled back the covers for a second time. Five minutes later, Steve and I hurried out the front door of our townhouse to the unattached garage. A two-foot-long icicle fell from the roof when I closed the door. The snow sparkled under the cold moonlit night.

Inside the garage, ice crystals coated everything, transforming the austere space into an ice palace. We got in the car and waited for it to warm up. Both of us sat hunched with our coats buttoned tight. Our legs tingled as we sat on the frozen leather seats of my little car.

"Did I ever tell you about the time I tried to shift the farm truck before it was ready?" I asked Steve.

"No," Steve's teeth rattled as he responded. He took off his gloves and blew into his hands in a desperate attempt to get warm.

In high school, I was an all-around on the gymnastics team. One especially cold night, I was in a hurry to get home after practice. I let the truck warm up just a few minutes and then shifted into drive. I heard a loud crack, and disaster struck. The handle snapped off in my hand, about an inch above where it connected to the column. Obviously, I did not warm up the truck long enough.

My Dad always left an assortment of tools in each vehicle. He said it was just in case something happened, but I often wondered if he just forgot them. I rummaged through the glove compartment and found a vice grip covered in rust. I placed the jaws around what was left of the shift handle and tightened down the flange on the top. It coated my fingers with brown dust. When the truck warmed up, I gingerly grabbed the handle and tried to shift. Much to my relief, the vice grip held. I drove home, proud of my creativity. Unfortunately, Dad did not share my enthusiasm. He made me pay for the repair.

On this equally frigid night, we warmed up the car and headed for the clinic. As we entered the parking lot, Steve spotted a Jeep parked in front. Salt and dirt covered the sides, and large accumulations of frozen slush hung behind each wheel. The vehicle's red color barely showed beneath all the grime. A 20-something man in a purple nylon jacket hopped out of the driver's side, ran to the passenger's side and removed a cat-sized carrier wrapped in a blanket.

Inside, Steve headed to the treatment room with a can of Moun-

tain Dew in his hand. He knew the drill by heart. I led Scott to the
cat exam room and flipped on the lights. It startled the fish resting
at the bottom of the tank. The poor guys were enjoying the fish
equivalent of sleep when I flooded the room in light. They swam
in erratic circles. "Sorry, guys," I said apologetically. I flipped off
the lights and escorted Scott to the dog room.

Genny meowed from her room. When she was 5 months old,
we moved her sleeping area from the bottom cage in the treatment
room to a spare storage room. The 12- by 8-foot space gave her
plenty of room to run and play. A covered litter box sat in the far
corner while the opposite one held her food and water bowl. In
between, toys littered the floor. Three different beds lined the walls.
Yes, Genny was spoiled. She preferred life that way.

Moe lay coiled in a tight ball amid his blankets and toys. He hid
his dark brown face, feet and tail in the champagne-colored fur of
his body. I talked to him in a soothing voice and gently jiggled his
blanket. Like Steve, ferrets are sound sleepers. They take awhile
to wake up from a deep sleep. I learned that lesson the hard way
when I picked up a sleeping ferret – I still have the bite marks on
my thumb to prove it.

"Moe, Moe," I cooed. "It's time to wake up." I reached into the
carrier and rubbed his back with my hand. The little ferret lifted
his head and yawned. He had a full set of sharp teeth. I stroked him
a few more times before picking him up.

Ferrets are pliable animals. Their ability to compress their
bodies to fit through tight spaces in search of prey comes in handy
for physical exams. If the ferret holds still, I can feel most of its
abdominal organs right through the skin. I held Moe's front end
with one hand and palpated his body with the other. When my fingers reached the small intestines, he squirmed. I placed him on the
blanket and tried again with a lighter touch. This time I felt a small,
firm, irregular-shaped foreign body next to the bladder.

"I'm afraid he swallowed a piece of the toy, Scott." I settled Moe
back on his blanket. "I can feel it right in the middle of his

abdomen." A piece this size was too large to pass through Moe's intestines. Surgery was the only option. Scott blew his long curly bangs out of his face and rubbed his hands together. His ears were still red from the cold.

"There's no other cheaper way to remove it?"

I shook my head. Scott thought for a moment. He loved his ferret but spent most of his paycheck going out every evening. I knew he customarily maxed out both of his credit cards just to cover the rent.

"Can I make payments? I don't have that kind of money on me right now."

I studied his face carefully before responding. I knew he loved the ferrets, but something about him made me question his integrity. He seemed a little slick, and besides, I was in no financial condition to get into the credit business. "Yes, as long as you put 30 percent down and pay the rest off within three months," I replied. Looking at the poor animal, I responded as vets too often do, from the heart, not the brain.

"No problem, I'll get a second job if I have to," he said.

Steve helped me take an X-ray of the ferret. I wanted to make sure I wasn't missing anything, especially in his chest. Sometimes, animals with something stuck in their esophagus will salivate excessively. Moe's chest looked good, but his intestines were distended with gas, which looked like big commas on the X-ray. Right in the middle of his abdomen, I spotted a gray-white mass.

I placed Moe's head in a clear plastic cone and turned on the anesthetic gas. Within minutes, he slept peacefully in my hands. With Steve's help, I passed an endotracheal tube down his windpipe. I tied the tube in place behind his ears and hooked it up to the anesthesia machine. Before I clipped the fur from the abdomen, I laid Moe on his side and clipped the hair from his front leg. Scott stood by my side, surprised by what he saw.

"What are you doing?" he asked quizzically. "The foreign body is in his abdomen."

"See that faint blue line?" I pointed at the cephalic vein on his forearm. "I'm going to try and place a catheter in that vein for fluids. He's really dehydrated." I scrubbed the leg and rinsed it with rubbing alcohol. Steve clamped his fingers around Moe's elbow. I could barely see the vein. I pumped his paw a few times. The blue line looked a little bigger, but this was going to be a challenge. I popped the tip of our smallest catheter through the skin and with a quick jab, pushed it into the vein. Bright red blood appeared in the hub of the needle. I slowly advanced it and slid off the catheter.

Steve handed me small pieces of white medical tape to hold the catheter in place. I attached a fluid line to it and opened the valve. Steve gave him a bolus of fluids to rehydrate him while I finished the abdominal clip.

We transferred Moe to the operating room and prepared him for surgery. Steve scrubbed the surgical site while I scrubbed my hands. Scott sat on a stool next to the operating table. He wore a bouffant cap over his hair and a mask over his nose and mouth. I backed into the room holding my hands in front of me. Water ran down my arms and dripped onto the floor from my elbows.

"Now Scott, if you feel at all queasy during this, tell us immediately. I do not want you to faint. OK?" I picked up a towel from the sterile pack. Scott had seen surgery before and assured me he wouldn't faint. "But that surgery wasn't on your own pet," I said. "Promise me you'll say something if you feel faint?" He nodded but seemed annoyed at my insistence.

I finished drying my hands on the blue surgical towel. Constant scrubbing for the O.R. dried out the skin on my hands. The low winter humidity didn't help, either. One deep crack on my thumb hurt every time I scrubbed. I picked up a sterile gown, held it by the ties and slid my hands down the sleeves, but not through them. Steve tied the straps on the back of the gown at my neck and waist. When we scrubbed with Lance, I found this romantic. Tonight, I was too tired to feel the spark. I put on a pair of gloves as I walked to the table.

In the background, the EKG beeped in regular rhythm. Steve

placed the large general pack on a Mayo stand. He pulled open the
wrapper one side at a time and folded it down around the stand.
Then, like the good O.R. nurse Lance had trained, he dropped a
series of drapes, sponges, suction tubing and flush onto the stand.
I placed the sterile drapes over Moe's body until only a small portion of his shaved abdomen was visible.

I nodded at Steve. He opened a shiny metal package over the
instruments. A 15 scalpel blade fell out and lodged in the handle
of a needle holder. I removed it, attached it to a scalpel handle and
made a three-inch incision down the center of Moe's abdomen.
Gas-distended loops of intestine bulged out of the incision. They
reminded me of the long balloons clowns use to make birthday
favors. I pushed them from side to side as I explored Moe's
abdomen. Everything felt great until I reached the intestines. About
halfway through the small bowel, I felt a firm object. The intestine
behind the object looked normal.

I pulled the area with the foreign body out of Moe's abdominal
cavity and packed it off with wet lap sponges. Leakage of intestinal
contents back into the cavity is one of the great threats encountered
in GI work. With everything in place, I incised just behind the toy
in the part of the intestine that looked normal. A small green piece
of plastic popped into my hand. I dropped it in a towel that Steve
placed on the counter.

Scott studied the object. "That's the leg and foot from one of
his toy dinosaurs. It's his favorite toy."

"Was his favorite," Steve corrected, now energized by Mountain
Dew.

I closed the incision in the intestine and rinsed Moe's abdomen
with copious amounts of sterile flush. Steve laid out a new pair of
sterile gloves. I struggled to change into those while he removed
the contaminated instruments from the table. During surgery, my
hands sweat in the gloves. The new ones stuck when I tried to pull
them on. Smile creases appeared on Steve's face under his mask.
"Do you need some help, Doctor?" he asked, emphasizing the word

Doctor.

"No, but you can drop the suture." I pulled the slack out of my gloves by pulling them tight over my fingertips. He pulled a pack of suture from his pocket. With both hands, he pulled the protective wrapper apart and dropped it to the stand. I grasped the needle with a Mayo-Hegar and began threading the suture through Moe's thin skin. For 10 minutes my hands moved back and forth over the incision. Using the plastic surgeon's technique, I buried the final layer under the skin to hide it from Moe's teeth. Ferrets are notorious for removing their sutures prematurely and without veterinary supervision.

Steve turned the big dial on the anesthesia vaporizer until it clicked at zero. I reached behind my back, untied the gown and pulled it off along with the gloves. Moe moved his lower jaw a little. His body started to shiver. A few seconds later, he swallowed. Steve pulled the tube from his throat. Moe coughed and sputtered.

"It's OK, little buddy," Scott said in a soothing voice. I unclipped the electrodes from the ferret's arms and legs, wrapped him in a towel and handed him to Scott. Moe blinked several times under the bright O.R. lights and yawned. He seemed better already. Scott ran his fingers over Moe's head. Back and forth, he stroked his pet. Moe closed his eyes and drifted off to sleep.

"Thanks for doing surgery on him, Kris, especially in the middle of the night. I really appreciate it," he said. I nodded and escorted him to the incubator in the treatment room. For Christmas, Steve bought me a used one from a human hospital. The temperature on the incubator read 88 degrees Fahrenheit. I pulled off my mask and cap and opened a portal into the chamber. "He's going to spend the day in here recovering."

Scott kissed his pet on the head and placed him in my powder-covered hands. I bunched the towels into a nest and laid Moe in the center. He looked around for five seconds, yawned again and then curled up into a tight ball. He soon closed his eyes and fell into a deep sleep. "Good night, little buddy," Scott whispered through the acrylic top. "Sweet dreams."

CHAPTER 15

Genevieve's Spay

After three hours of sleep, I returned to the clinic with a pounding headache. My head ached with each step, feeling like it would explode. I walked around the counter without a word. The only thing on my mind was sleep. I scanned the appointment book in hope of finding time for a nap. Names scribbled in pencil filled most of the morning slots. A big X with the word "surgery" crossed out all the appointments from noon until 2.

"What have we got for surgery?"

"Two spays, Genny and Chiffon Cummings," Allie answered.

"I thought a specialist would spay Chiffon when they took care of her other problems?"

"That was the plan," Allie confirmed. Evidently, Chiffon did so well on the lactulose that her owner postponed the other surgery. The little furball was Julie Cummings' constant companion. She only left her owner's bed to eat, drink or go outside. The pup grew into a four-pound guard dog who kept an eye on all the people coming and going. No one could touch the young woman without passing a sniff test. Under Chiffon's care, Julie's physical condition and attitude improved. Chiffon gave Julie a reason to live.

"How is Moe doing today?" I asked as I unbuttoned my thick winter jacket.

"Great, I didn't see any vomitus in the incubator." Allie handed me a stack of messages. "But you forgot to give him a litter box." She smiled at me as she recalled the details. Moe jumped into the litter and started to urinate without even digging a hole. "The poor guy really had to go."

By the time I finished the stack of messages, the waiting room bustled with people and animals. Two golden retriever puppies needed their booster shots. A diabetic cat needed a glucose check. Winston needed his anal glands expressed again. The morning flew by. Before we knew it, the clock read 12:30, and neither of us had eaten anything.

"Allie," I called as she headed to the lobby with a bottle of pink amoxicillin. "I'll get us lunch if you set up the O.R. for Chiffon and Genny. Steve has a client meeting in Burnsville this afternoon. He's going to stop by after the meeting." I pulled my winter coat off the hook in the closet. "I want her done before he arrives."

Allie knew how protective Steve was of his little princess. It would be in everyone's best interest to finish her before he arrived. She nodded and shook the bottle in her hand. "I'll take care of this client, then work on the O.R."

Fifteen minutes later, I returned to the clinic with two sandwiches. Allie stood at the front counter, her ear glued to the phone and an annoyed expression on her face. "OK, then, bring her right in," she said in a reluctant voice before she hung up the phone. "Sorry, Dr. Nelson, but we have an emergency coming in."

Great, I thought to myself between bites of lunch. We'll never get Genny done before Steve arrives.

We hadn't finished eating when the doorbell rang. In walked a couple, Helen and Timothy Johnson with their young son, Robert, and daughter, Alison. She cradled a brown tabby cat in a blanket. The anxious parents stood at the counter while the kids took a seat in the waiting room. The little girl buried her face in the blanket and cried. Allie quickly ushered the family into the cat exam room.

"Dr. Nelson, we think Ariel broke her back," the father said. "My son fell on her and ..."

"I did not fall on her," Robert interrupted his father. His mother jerked her head toward him and gave him a look that brought immediate silence.

"Robert, I told you not to lie," she scolded.

"I'm not lying. You don't believe me." He turned around and faced the aquarium with both hands on his hips.

"Sorry about that, Dr. Nelson," the man continued. "We were packing for a trip when we noticed Ariel lying on the floor with her back in a strange position. Then she started to cry." He looked at the cat in his daughter's arms. "She's in horrible pain."

I looked at the information sheet the couple filled out. Ariel was a present for Alison's 7th birthday. She was 8 weeks old back then, so she must be about 9 months old now. Ariel had received all her kitten shots but was not spayed.

"OK, please put Miss Ariel on the table for me. Let's see what's wrong with her."

When I removed the blanket, Ariel yawned, rolled onto her side and stretched her entire body. Her brown tabby stripes ended in brown spots on her tummy. She was a beautiful girl with long graceful legs and a fluffy tail. I petted her head and then ran my hand over her back. Ariel scrambled to her feet. She thrust her rear end high into the air but kept her chest on the ground like she was praying. When I scratched her back just in front of her tail, she yowled and closed her eyes.

"That's what she's been doing, Dr. Nelson," the man said. The couple exchanged worried glances.

"And rolling around on the floor, too," the woman added. "The poor thing is in pain."

I tried not to burst out laughing. "She is in pain," I said in a soothing voice. "But it is not the kind of pain you think it is." The parents looked at me quizzically as I continued the exam. Ariel reveled in the attention. She flopped from one side to the other and meowed when I hit a good spot. There was just one last item to check before announcing the diagnosis.

"OK, I need to take her temperature."

"Honey, hold onto her for this," Helen instructed her husband. As a kitten at her exam, she had hated this, leaving two long scratch marks on Helen's arm. Timothy placed both hands on Ariel and braced for the worst.

"I don't think you have to worry about being scratched today." I shot a wry smile at the couple while I covered the end of the thermometer with lube. I scratched the magic spot just in front of her tail. She raised her rear end high in the air. The minute the tip of the thermometer touched her skin, she froze in place. A strange look of contentment spread over her face. She relaxed her ears to the side and closed her eyes. As the seconds ticked by on my watch, Ariel purred and purred. I removed the thermometer. Timothy relaxed his grip.

"Wow, are you ever good, Dr. Nelson," Helen said. "She was awful the last time." I smiled and nodded my head.

"So what do you think is wrong with Ariel?" Timothy couldn't wait any longer.

I thought for a moment before I responded. "Ariel is in heat." I looked straight into the couple's eyes. They looked at each other, clearly confused by this turn of events.

"That can't be," Helen replied. "She's not even a year old yet. She's just a baby."

"Well, your baby has grown up." I smiled. "Cats may go into heat anytime after 6 months of age. It's common for spring and summer kittens to have their first heat in January."

"But she's rolling around in pain," Timothy countered, not ready to believe me.

"That is normal behavior for a cat in heat," I responded. "The hormones make them act that way." Silence filled the room as the couple pondered the situation. Timothy petted Ariel. She continued to roll around on the table.

After a minute, the little boy turned his attention from the angelfish to me. "What is heat?" he asked. Helen's eyes widened. Timothy blushed. They looked at each other but were at a loss for words.

"Heat means Ariel is growing up from a baby kitten to an adult cat," I answered with a smile on my face. I bit my lip to keep from laughing.

"Oh," he said, and returned his attention to the fish tank. Helen's eyes returned to their normal size and the bright red color left her husband's face.

"Are you sure about this?" Timothy asked. "I mean ..." he paused. "She seems so pained."

I leaned forward and whispered. "As a vet, I can tell you the only time a cat enjoys having its temperature taken is when it is in heat." Instantly, his face turned red again. Helen gasped and started to laugh. As often happens with guys, Timothy was clearly uncomfortable. He was relieved the cat was OK, but at this point looked for any opportunity to get out of the clinic.

Alison could not understand her parent's reaction. After studying all the adults for a moment, she blurted out a very important question. "Will Ariel be alright?"

"Ariel will be fine," I answered in as reassuring a voice as I could muster. "Now that she has grown into a mature cat, she needs to be spayed." I looked at the parents. "Otherwise she will keep going in and out of heat until she ..." I paused searching for a nice way to say get pregnant. "Until her needs are satisfied."

"You got to be kidding," Timothy said. Helen burst into laughter again – big heaving belly laughs that left her with tears in her eyes.

"No, I'm afraid I'm not," I replied. "They act like this for a week or so, relax for a few days and start again." Helen stopped laughing long enough to wipe the tears from her checks. Her husband's face turned an even deeper shade of red. "You know how much noise the stray cats make at night," I said. They both nodded. "That's what you're in for unless you spay her."

"Well, we were planning on taking her with us," Timothy responded.

"We're going to Iowa to see Grandma and Grandpa," Robert chimed in.

I suggested they leave Ariel at the clinic during their trip. We could spay her tomorrow and then let her recuperate in the hospital. By the time the family returned, she would be back to normal, her days of raging hormones over.

"That sounds great to me," Timothy responded. "What do you think, honey?"

A look of sadness filled his wife's eyes. "I planned to let Ariel have one litter to let the kids experience the miracle of life." She patted her daughter's shoulder. "I thought it would be a wonderful thing to share as a family."

As I veterinarian, I hear this a lot. Women who experience the miracle of life want to share it with their children. They believe it will be one of those memories the family can share forever. Unfortunately, these moms often have no idea what they are in for. I work hard to give them the facts necessary to make an informed decision.

First, I discussed the problem of finding a mate for Ariel. Since no reputable breeder would let their purebred tom breed with a shelter cat, their options were limited. They could find a friend with an intact male pet or let Ariel go outside in search of love. But this would expose Ariel to all kinds of dangers from infectious disease, being attacked by a dog or hit by a car. The second problem was Ariel's size. Because she was petite, an emergency C-section might be needed to deliver the kittens. A C-section is not inexpensive surgery. Third, finding good homes for the offspring is a lot of work. To complicate matters further, cats usually give birth at night. Families often endure the work only to miss the birth.

Before I could continue, Helen raised her hand with the palm facing me. "OK, I get the point." She looked at her husband. "I agree. Let's get her spayed while we're gone." I breathed a sigh of relief. With all the unwanted animals in the world, I felt great about preventing more. I picked up Ariel and cuddled her against my face. A worried look spread over the little girl's face, tears welled in her eyes.

In a nod to Dr. Anderson of my youth I said, "Would you like to come in back and see where Ariel is going to stay?" Alison slowly nodded her head and grabbed her mother's hand. "Robert, would you like to come as well?" He nodded and put his hand on her purse. "OK then, follow me." I escorted the family through the pharmacy into the treatment room. I opened the door to a cage above Scruffy's former abode.

"May we keep her blanket so she has something from home to comfort her?" I asked. Alison nodded. She folded the blanket into a neat square and placed it in the cage.

"What's wrong with that cat?" Robert pointed at Genny. She slept in the cage next to Ariel.

"Nothing," I replied. "She is going to be spayed today. We gave her a tranquilizer to calm her down. It makes them sleepy." The little boy nodded. His head barely reached the second tier of cages. "We'll do the same with Ariel," I added.

One by one, Helen, Alison and Robert hugged Ariel. When they finished, I placed her in the cage and latched the door. Allie escorted them out while I changed into scrubs. The clock read 1 p.m. Steve was expected around 2:30.

Chiffon went first. I spayed her and also removed the baby teeth in record time. Then it was Genny's turn. Under the effect of the tranquilizer, her precocious attitude disappeared. Through the wonders of pharmaceuticals, Genny was transformed into a model patient. Within minutes she slept under the bright lights of the surgery table. Her heart beat in a regular rhythm. I left to scrub my hands in the prep sink while Allie scrubbed Genny's tummy.

After Allie tied the gown behind my back, I slipped on a pair of sterile gloves. The clock read 1:50. There should be plenty of time to finish before Steve arrived. Sitting on a stool by Genny's head,

Allie slipped her hand under the drapes to feel Genny's heart and looked at the EKG.

I got right to work. After draping off the surgical area, I incised her abdomen. I inserted a long instrument with a hook at the end into the incision. The spay hook made it much easier to grab the ovaries and uterus. When I pulled it back out, Genny's left ovary lay inside. There's nothing like finding it on the first try. I ligated the ovarian pedicle, removed the ovary and moved to the other side. Again, the right ovary popped into view on the first try.

With the hardest part over, I moved to the uterus. In cats, the uterus is a small Y shaped organ. The arms of the Y are very long while the body is short. This allows the queen to carry multiple fetuses with ease. I ligated the uterus just above the cervix and removed it along with the ovaries from Genny's abdomen. Before closing, I peeked inside one more time.

"She looks good. I'm closing now." Allie nodded and made a note on her clipboard. With only the incision left, I felt confident that we'd finish before Steve arrived. I grabbed a needle holder and suture from the Mayo stand. The needle passed in and out of the muscles with ease. Allie stood up to view the incision.

"I'm turning her off," she said. I continued to work, with the needle moving in and out of Genny's skin.

"Ding, ding" the doorbell sounded. Allie looked at her watch. It read 2:05. She put down her clipboard. "Are you OK so I can see who it is?" I nodded.

Before she could leave, Steve's face appeared in the window. He looked concerned. He had raced to the clinic to check on his precious Genny. Allie and I looked at each other and shrugged. He cracked opened the door.

"Hi, Allie, hi, Krissy, who are you working on? I didn't see Genny in the cages."

I responded with my eyes still trained on the incision. "I'm finishing Genny's spay. You're early."

"Yes, the meeting ended early. I rushed to get here as fast as I could," he announced with pride. I threaded the suture just below the surface of Genny's skin.

"Are you doing the plastic-surgeon closure?" Steve asked. "I know Genny will chew out sutures in her skin."

Allie looked at me and rolled her eyes. Before I could answer, he asked Allie if she was bagging her at regular intervals. Allie nodded and to emphasize the point squeezed the black bag attached to the oxygen machine. Fresh gas rushed through the system.

"She's all done." I released the towel clamps and rolled the drapes into a ball. Allie loosened the ties on her front legs while I released the ones on her back legs. With that done, she unclipped the leads to the EKG. For two minutes, Genny breathed pure oxygen from the machine before she started to cough. Allie pulled the trach tube out of her mouth. She coughed twice more, then relaxed. I swaddled her tight in a towel with only her face showing. She continued to sleep as the anesthetic wore off.

"Here's our little princess, dear," I said to Steve. I walked into the treatment room with Genny in my arms, holding her on her back like a human baby.

"Oh, poor little Genevieve. She looks so precious." He petted her head and kissed her forehead. He extended his arms toward me. "I'll hold her while she wakes up."

"I don't think that's a good idea, dear." I tried to discourage him. Some cats wake up having nightmares. They growl and bite at imaginary monsters. They do much better in a quiet cage without any stimulation.

"No, I want to hold her. She'll be fine with her Dad." He left me no choice. I handed Genny over to him. He flipped his tie over his shoulder and held her close to his chest. "We'll be in the office," he announced and left the room. I removed the cap from my head and fluffed my hair with both hands.

"Where's Genny?" Allie asked when she returned from the O.R., carrying the surgical instruments rolled up in a drape.

"She's in the office. Steve wants to hold her as she recovers."

Allie looked surprised. "I know," I said, pulling the mask from my neck. "I'll keep an eye on them."

Steve sat in the middle of the office on a folding chair. Genny slept in his arms, still wrapped in the blanket. I made phone calls just outside the door. Steve rocked our little bundle back and forth in his arms and motioned for me to turn off the office lights. He felt they were too bright for her eyes. With that, Steve took control of the recovery. She was definitely Daddy's little girl.

I dialed the first number. Beep, beep, beep, the line was busy. I placed the note at the bottom on the stack. I dialed the next number. Just as it started to ring, I heard a loud growl from inside the office. I slammed the receiver down and returned to the office. Genny looked possessed. Her eyes were huge, seeing all kinds of scary monsters. Steve pressed her against his chest as he struggled to keep her under control. The growls grew louder and more ferocious by the second. She managed to get her one rear leg out of the towel. Her tail whipped Steve's leg.

"Steve, give her to me," I commanded. Undeterred, he continued to rock back and forth, ignoring me. "Steve, now!" I yelled. As he tried to comply, Genny freed herself from the towel. She pinned her ears flat against her head and hissed at Steve. Her eyes were open, but she didn't recognize him. A split second later, she jumped at his face with her teeth bared and claws out.

I grabbed her by the scruff of the neck just before she made contact with his face. She twisted her body and took a swipe at me with her front claws. I held her at arm's length and ran to the treatment room. Allie opened a cage door. I dropped her inside and slammed the door behind her. She spun around and swiped at me again.

"Are you OK?" Allie asked. I nodded. "Caught her in midair." I panted from the excitement. "She was going to rip Steve's face off." Genny uttered a long, low growl from the recesses of her cage. All the hair on her back and tail stood on end. She hissed and charged the front of the cage. Allie and I jumped back in unison.

That was a close one, too close for comfort. Allie blew a stray hair out of her face and covered the front of the cage with a towel. Most cats calm down in a dark space.

I returned to Steve, who sat frozen in the same position as when I left him. "I can't believe she did that to me," he said to himself more than to me. "She's known me since she was a day-old kitten. I fed her." He looked at me with a pathetic expression on his face. "I even cleaned her rear end."

I placed my hand on his shoulder. "It's the drugs, dear. I told you some cats, especially ones with her attitude, wake up hallucinating." My words were of no comfort. He wrung his hands together. "And who knows what she saw ... a nasty dog, a monster or maybe Scruffy." I waited for a laugh, but Steve did not respond. He started to emerge from the shock. I made him promise that he would never try to hold another cat during recovery.

Steve stood up and put his arm around my shoulder. "Yes, dear," he replied.

Allie appeared in the doorway with good news. Covering the cage worked great. Genny now slept peacefully. Steve readjusted his tie, put on his long wool winter coat and picked up his briefcase.

"Hey, Allie, I keep forgetting to ask about Scruffy. How's he doing?"

"I saw him over Christmas. He's huge. You wouldn't recognize him." The best news of all is that he stopped knocking things off the counter. Mike played with him so much he was too tired to get into trouble.

"I'm glad to hear that he's doing well." Steve smiled at me. "Well, I better get back to work. Now that I've taken care of Genny, I'll leave her in your hands."

"Don't you mean that Genny has taken care of you?" I couldn't resist.

"I'll see you at home," he said. He pulled the car keys out of a pocket and kissed me on the cheek.

CHAPTER 16

Butch the Alpha Pup

"Dr. Nelson, your next appointment is a new puppy exam." Allie smiled as she handed me the chart. "The little guy already weighs 30 pounds, and he's only 8 weeks old."

I knocked on the solid door, two sharp raps to alert my clients inside before entering. A 30-something man sat in a chair on the opposite site of the room. A black pup with a white crest on his chest lay at his feet. The pup looked up at me while savoring the bootlace in his mouth.

After introducing myself to Dan Arnold, I greeted the Great Dane. "And you must be Butch." The puppy looked up at me without releasing the bootlace. The excess skin on his forehead wrinkled into rows that reminded me of a plowed field. He thumped his tail twice before focusing on the other boot. "Before I examine Butch, I need to ask a few questions," I said. The man nodded.

Dan purchased Butch from a Great Dane breeder south of the Twin Cities. The kennel's contract required a veterinary examination within 48 hours of purchase. If the new owner failed to comply, the contract stipulated the kennel would not be responsible for any health problems discovered at a later date. Having paid more than $1,000, the man took the afternoon off work to make sure the pup was healthy.

"Has he been vaccinated and dewormed?" I asked. Dan pulled a crumpled paper from the back pocket of his blue jeans. He ran it back and forth over the arm of the chair to remove the wrinkles before handing it to me. As I studied it, Butch wandered around the exam room. Bored with shoelaces, he looked for something new to chew on. He crawled under the man's chair and emerged on the other side with dust bunnies on his face.

According to the document, Butch needed another booster shot today. He also needed a fecal check for parasites. I made a quick note in the chart and handed the paper back to Dan.

"The breeder already wormed him," the new owner replied. "I'm not made of money, ya know." Here it comes, I thought.

I explained that while it was true that the breeder gave Butch three doses of a puppy de-wormer, there was no record of a fecal analysis. Without the test, there was no way to know if Butch had intestinal parasites. He could have been given an unnecessary drug. In addition, there is no perfect de-worming medicine guaranteed to remove every parasite. Without identifying a specific one, the breeder was just shotgunning.

Silence hung over the room as I waited for a response. Dan gazed at me without blinking. Creases appeared around his eyes; his weathered skin made him look much older than he really was. "The technician mentioned something about heartworms. Will this test for that, too?"

I explained that heartworms actually live in the heart, so a fecal check, which finds parasites living in the gastrointestinal tract, would not identify them. Mosquitoes transmit juvenile heartworms from animal to animal with the bite. The immature worm swims to the heart and matures into an adult – hence the name heartworm. Every year, we take a sample of blood to check for this parasite.

Since Butch was a pup, he would begin heartworm prevention right away without the test. Once a month, he'd think he was getting a treat.

"I wanna get Butch everything he needs. I have big plans for him."

"Errrrrrrh," the pup cried. He lay on the floor with his nose pressed into the crack between the door and the threshold. His nostrils flared. When nothing happened, he scratched the door with one paw before looking up at us. Something smelled really good on the other side.

"I think he agrees," I responded.

"I'm gonna use him as a stud dog," the man said, looking into my eyes with a smile on his face. "He comes from champions, you know."

"Wow, congratulations." The hard part for an experienced vet faced with this news is to sound genuinely amazed. Every new owner of a pup registered with the American Kennel Club regales me with this statement.

"Alright, Butch, it's time for your exam. Please put him on the table, Mr. Arnold."

"Call me Dan." The man placed one hand under Butch's chest and another around his rear end. "Come, buddy. It's time to see the doctor." He lifted him up onto the table and sat himself down again.

"Hi, handsome," I cooed. Butch looked up at me from the middle of the table. He seemed uncomfortable on the slippery surface. "Let's take a peek at you." I placed my hands on the top of his head and rubbed his neck. Butch wagged his tail and reached up to lick my lips. I turned my face to the side, allowing the pup to lick my chin instead. The unmistakable smell of puppy breath washed over my face.

I lifted up each ear and peered into the canals. Butch sat still until I inserted the tip of the otoscope into his left ear. He spun his head around and gave me a warning look.

"Would you mind putting a hand on him for this?" I asked the owner. Dan rose from the chair.

"You hold still, Butch." The pup looked at him, then allowed me to thoroughly examine his ears, eyes and nose. I pried open his mouth with my fingers. Baby teeth with sharp points lined the upper and lower jaws. Pieces of dog chow stuck in the corners of his mouth. All of the teeth meshed with each other in perfect occlusion. Now my hands also smelled like puppy breath.

"So far, so good," I stated and removed the stethoscope from my neck. I cleaned a piece of fur from one of the tips before placing them in my ears. Butch leaned forward. He placed his mouth around the metal bell and tubing of the instrument. "Oh no, you don't," I said. I removed it from his powerful jaws and placed it on his chest, right behind the left front leg. The scarred tubing, no match for sharp teeth or strong beaks, reminded me of other close calls with dogs, cats and birds. My last stethoscope only lasted a year before a parrot sliced it in half. With my tight budget, I hoped this one would last longer.

"Lub, dub. Lub, dub." The sounds echoed in my ears. "Lub, dub, lub, dub." His rhythm was regular and strong. "Lub dub. Lub dub." Each beat sounded sharp, no whooshes or clicks to indicate a problem. I replaced the stethoscope around my neck and motioned for Butch to stand. Dan hoisted the pup to his feet. The pup grunted and tried to sit down again. "Point his rear end toward me please," I instructed.

I placed both of my hands on Butch's abdomen and applied light pressure with my fingertips, just enough to feel the organs below. Because Great Danes have large chests, they're prone to an emergency condition called bloat. To prevent it, I advised Dan to feed several small meals per day as opposed to one big one that distends the stomach. I also recommended no exercise for at least one hour after eating. Dan nodded with squinted eyes. I continued to probe Butch's abdomen with my hands. "His spleen feels good, but he's got a lot of gas in his intestines."

"What does that mean?" Dan asked in a concerned voice.

"Well, it could be normal for him. It could also mean that he's got worms, or his food doesn't agree with him."

"I'll bring in a fecal sample as soon as I can." I smiled, amused by his changed perspective.

My right hand moved back to Butch's scrotum. It sounds elementary, but one of the most important aspects of a purchase exam is to confirm that both testicles are present. During development, one or both testicles may become trapped inside the abdomen, a condition called cryptorchidism. Dogs with this condition are disqualified from the show ring. I felt two large symmetrical testicles in the scrotum. "But I'm glad to tell you that Butch has all of his equipment."

I studied Dan's expression. I don't read all men correctly, but Dan seemed like the type who would appreciate acknowledgment of his dog's male virtues. "And I must say, he is very well endowed." A huge smile spread over the owner's face. He patted the pup's side with pride oozing from every pore. I don't know why this matters so much to guys, but it makes their day when I offer a distinguished medical opinion that their dog is a stud. I finished the exam by flexing both of Butch's hips and knees.

"Just a quick vaccination, and you're done," I said.

"I want to get his ears fixed," Dan stated. "Do you do that, Doc?"

"No, I don't." I squeezed a few drops of rubbing alcohol onto the skin over his right shoulder. "I'm not a fan of ear cropping. I think he looks great just the way God made him."

"But I want to get them done so I can show him," Dan replied.

"Then I would call the breeder for a recommendation. I don't know of any veterinarians who perform ear crops." I handed a dog biscuit to Dan. "Do not give it to him until I tell you to. Just let him sniff it." I retrieved a syringe filled with pink solution from the drawer beneath the counter, held it upright and flicked the side with my finger. Air bubbles collected in the neck of the syringe. I pushed the plunger in, releasing a pink mist into the air.

"Are you ready?" I asked. Dan nodded. "Show him the cookie." While Butch sniffed the cookie, I moved the syringe toward his skin. "OK, Dan." I scratched the skin with my fingernail. As Dan handed him the biscuit, I pierced Butch's skin with the syringe.

"Grrrrrrrl," a deep growl emanated from the pup, illustrating that the vocal cords were in fine order. The biscuit fell out of his mouth onto the table. I jumped back, pulling the needle out of his skin but failing to inject any vaccine. Young pups often cry when I vaccinate them, but I never had one growl.

"Knock it off," I ordered. Butch looked up at me without blinking. I returned his stare. For a full minute, the two of us stood frozen in time, staring at each other, neither of us willing to submit. "Your pup needs an attitude adjustment," I whispered to Dan without looking away. "If it's OK with you, I'm going to show him that I'm the boss by holding him on his back until he looks away."

"No, I like his attitude. I don't want no wimp at my house," the owner said.

"You don't understand, Dan. Butch growled at me." My eyes remained locked with the puppy. "That's a bad sign. We need to nip this behavior in the bud while he's small. With the size he'll have, he could turn into a real monster." I held Butch's gaze as I spoke. "Please let me show you some techniques for improving his attitude."

"Ah, alright," Dan stammered. I put down the vaccine and placed both of my hands on Butch without looking away. In one quick motion, I pinned him on his back on the exam table. Butch struggled for several minutes. Loud growls rattled from his throat. His body thumped the table as his legs flailed in the air.

"No," I ordered. "No!" My hands ached as I continued to hold him on his back. His front leg caught the bell of the stethoscope and ripped it off my neck. It flew through the air and crashed to the floor.

"Let him go," Dan said.

"Not until he gives up," I grunted in reply. My back ached as well. "I cannot let go until he looks away." I could feel Dan's glare on the back of my head.

I continued to stand over the pup, staring into his eyes. After three minutes, Butch relaxed and finally looked away. "Good boy," I exclaimed releasing my grip from his neck. He rolled over and panted. "Good boy," I repeated. I scratched his back and looked at Dan. In pack behavior, staring is considered a provocative act. If Butch behaved like this with an adult pack member, the dog would grab him by the throat and pin him to the ground to teach respect. If Butch still refused to submit, he would face more serious consequences.

I rotated my shoulders and stretched my fingers. "Now let's try this again."

Dan stood next to the exam table. Butch snuggled into him without making eye contact with me. Again, I cleaned his skin with alcohol. "Ready?"

Dan nodded as he put his arm around Butch. "Let 'er rip."

I pulled the cap off the needle. With my left hand, I grasped the skin over the pup's right shoulder. On command, Dan gave Butch a biscuit. With my right hand, I pushed the needle through the skin. Butch turned his head toward me. A piece of cookie fell on the table. I stared back and shouted "No!" He looked away, and I injected the vaccine without incident. When the biscuit was gone, he nuzzled Dan's hand for more.

"Sorry pal, you ate them all." Dan started to lift him off the table.

"Wait a minute. I want to play with him a little to make this a good experience." Dan stepped back from the table. I placed another dog biscuit in front of the pup. He studied my face for a minute before sniffing the treat. "It's OK, handsome." I smiled and scratched him on the rump with both hands. Small pieces of dandruff rose to the surface of his coat. I smoothed the hair and brushed them off.

Butch grabbed the treat. Two chomps later, it was gone. He licked the table, leaving a wet patch where the treat rested. "See, it's not so bad to come to the vet." I cradled his head in my hands and looked into his big brown eyes. "You get lots of treats." Butch glanced briefly at me before turning his attention to Dan. I scratched him again and placed him on the ground.

"When do we have to come back?" Dan clipped the leash onto Butch's collar and put his hand on the doorknob.

"He needs another vaccination in three weeks." I put the pup's chart on the table. "And I want you to start obedience training with him right away. He needs to learn that he is not the boss."

Dan smiled and opened the door. "We'll see you in three weeks."

CHAPTER 17

Puppy Hit by Car

March in Minnesota is a tease. After months of darkness and cold, Minnesotans are ready for winter to end. Warm sun melts snow into slushy piles. Patches of dried grass appear here and there. At 5:30 p.m., the sky is still light enough to drive home in daylight. A zillion degrees below zero gives way to the balmy 30s. People leave their hats and scarves at home, reveling in the warm temperatures. Then, insidiously, the temperature plummets as an arctic air mass descends from Canada.

During an especially warm day, Butch returned with Dan for his second set of shots. The pup walked into the clinic with each ear bandaged into a tight roll. They flopped back and forth with each step. Butch weighed in at a hefty 46 pounds. His feet were enormous; they didn't fit his body. He left muddy footprints the size of a saucer all over our waiting room.

Due to his behavior during our first encounter, I took extra time with Butch during this visit. I used a chew toy to distract him throughout the physical. Before the vaccination, I looked into Butch's eyes and rolled him on to his side to re-establish my authority. He glanced at me for a few seconds before deciding to submit.

So far, things were going well. I gave Dan some cookies and prepared the syringe. Butch ignored the cookies. He studied my every motion with an intensity that made me uncomfortable. He did not take his eyes off of me. When I reached for his shoulder with the rubbing alcohol container, Butch looked into my eyes for a brief second before turning away. I wasn't sure if he was acknowledging me as superior or simply sizing me up for later. He remained still when I injected the vaccine.

"Butch is going to be a big boy, even by Great Dane standards," I told Dan. As I rubbed the area where I had injected the vaccine, the puppy continued to watch me. On the table, his head was almost even with mine. "How's his training coming?"

"Great, he hasn't had an accident in over two weeks. I caught him peeing on the carpet once and that was it." Dan grinned from ear to ear. "He's a smart pup."

"That's great," I replied. I pushed a cookie toward Butch. He sniffed it, looked at me for a second and then gobbled it down. "How about obedience training? Did you enroll him in puppy kindergarten?"

"No need to." Dan grunted as he placed Butch on the ground. "I've been working with him at home. He minds me just fine." Butch ambled over to the door and looked up at us. Dan took a leather leash out of his pocket. "Butch, come here and let me hook you up." The pup stayed by the door and looked up at the handle. Dan walked over to him and clipped the leash to his collar.

"Dan, I know I sound like a broken record, but you really need to get him into obedience training. Besides teaching him basic commands, the classes will help socialize him with other people and animals. It's critical for giant-breed dogs to get good training as pups when you can still control them."

A wry smile spread over Dan's face as I talked. When I finished, he placed his hand on the doorknob and cracked the door open.

Butch pushed his face into the opening and forced the door wide open. "I'll see you again in three weeks, Doc," Dan said as the two left the room. The pair walked past a Miniature schnauzer sitting with a retired woman. The dog barked and then ran under a chair. Dan laughed before he pulled Butch out the front door. I headed to the back to finish writing up his medical record.

"Help, I need help!" a lady screamed from the front lobby. "My dog has been hit by a car." I recognized Jennifer Thomas' voice immediately. Dropping my pen, I ran toward the lobby.

"Jennifer, what ..." I froze in place. Jennifer stood in the middle of the lobby holding Captain's limp body in her arms. Blood poured down her pant leg onto the floor. Captain looked dead. The waiting client clasped both hands to her mouth in horror. Her dog sniffed the air and froze, seeming to sense the gravity of the situation.

"Bring him here," I ordered. She followed me through the clinic to the treatment room. I held Captain's head in my hands as Jennifer laid him on the table.

When Jennifer stepped back, I saw the source of the blood. The skin and hair on the outside of Captain's right front leg were gone, ripped away by the car. I could see bone, muscles and tendons. Blood drops collected on the underside of his leg like icicles on the edge of a roof and dripped into a large puddle on the floor.

"Oh, my God," Jennifer wailed when she looked at the injury. "Captain, Captain, please don't die!"

I grabbed a tourniquet from the drawer and slipped it over the bloody front leg. When it rested above the elbow, I cinched it into place. The dripping blood slowed to a trickle. The clock on the wall read 5:35 p.m. The tourniquet could stay in place for 40 minutes before Captain's leg suffered damage from the lack of blood flow. Time was of the essence.

"Allie, give me a bag of saline and a catheter setup," I said softly. "I'll prep for the cath." I pulled a clipper off the shelf, unwound the cord wrapped around it and plugged it in. As I shaved the dog's leg, black fur fell to the ground. Captain's gums were almost white, and his chest heaved up and down with every breath. I splashed alcohol over the vein. Captain did not have time for meticulous sterile prep. Allie plugged an extension set into a bag of clear fluids, hung it from a ceiling hook and evacuated air from the line. She grasped Captain's left elbow and held off the vein, which failed to swell because of the blood loss. Captain was in hemorrhagic shock. Allie flashed me a worried look.

I took the cap off the catheter, felt the leg one more time and thrust the tip into where I thought the vein should be. We watched the hub, but no flash of blood appeared. I hunched over and waited for it. Two precious seconds ticked by. The worried look on Allie's face intensified. I continued to watch the hub of the catheter. Since Captain's blood pressure was negligible, it would take longer for blood to flow into the catheter. If this didn't work, I would have to cut open his skin for direct visualization. I pumped his paw again. Much to my relief, a small amount of blood flashed into the hub of the catheter.

"You're in!" Allie exclaimed. I advanced the catheter a little farther into the vein and taped it to his leg in record time. As Allie opened the valve on the drip set all the way, clear fluid shot into his leg. Then she placed an oxygen mask over Captain's muzzle. In blood, the majority of the oxygen is carried on the red blood cells. A small amount diffuses into the plasma, the liquid part of blood. Giving Captain 100 percent oxygen to breathe would saturate his plasma and the red blood cells he had left.

I needed to check for arrhythmias. We clipped a wire lead from the EKG, which measures electrical impulses that spread through the heart, to each of Captain's legs. At first, the electronic tracing was hard to read. It bounced all over the screen every time Captain breathed. I fiddled with the position knob until visible waves crossed the screen. Captain's rate was fast, but so far there were no abnormal rhythms.

With the blood loss stopped and the catheter in, I stepped back to re-evaluate the situation. Jennifer lay over Captain's chest. Blood covered her face, glasses, shirt and pants. She was a sickly green. Her back heaved up and down in silent sobs.

"It's my fault. It's my fault," she wailed. "We were out walking, and the leash slipped out of my hand. I should have slipped it around my arm. It's my fault."

How do you comfort a pet owner in a situation like this? Telling them it was an accident rings hollow when the pet is fighting for its life. "Is your son OK?" I asked. She nodded.

"Blake is with his Dad this week." Jennifer's tears mixed with the blood on her face and left streaks down her cheeks. "It was my fault."

"Jennifer, he's getting better. See, he's not breathing so hard." I motioned toward Captain's chest. "Now, I want you to go with Allie and clean up." Allie took Jennifer by the arm and pulled her off Captain. More tears flowed down Jennifer's cheeks. Allie half escorted and half dragged her to the bathroom.

The clock on the wall read 5:45 p.m. when Allie returned to the treatment room. She caressed Captain's head and looked at the horrible wound on his leg. While she was away, the dog's color had improved from white to pale pink. His breaths came easier. Then Captain looked over the oxygen mask at Allie and thumped his tail twice. She caressed him again. "Can you save the leg?" she asked.

"I don't know. I need to clean this up and get a better look." Before we started to clip the leg, I gave Captain a dose of meperidine to ease the pain. Allie folded a towel and placed it under Captain's head. The poor dog closed his eyes and relaxed.

"Let's get going on this leg," I said. Allie hung another bag of fluids to flush the leg. While I donned a pair of surgical gloves, she threw a towel on the floor under Captain's leg. She rolled up another one and placed it between the dog's front legs to separate them. Next, she squeezed a large amount of sterile lube into the wound. This would keep the hair from sticking to the area.

Allie pushed the clipper through the hair. Large hunks fell onto the towel. The clipper groaned each time it hit a clump of dried blood. The blood gummed up the blade and made it stick to the fur and skin. Allie cleaned it out with a brush and sprayed the blade with clipper lube.

With the hair removed, we could see the full extent of Captain's wound. The skin on the right side of his leg was missing from the elbow down past the wrist, almost to his paw. The wound gapped open from the front of his leg all the way around to the back side. The edges were smooth, as if cut by a knife. Chunks of muscle were missing on the outside of the leg. Toward the wrist, I could see clear down to the bone. Pebbles, sand and road grit littered the wound.

Allie loosened the tourniquet a little and blood started to ooze from the damaged leg. One by one, I traced the leaks to damaged vessels, isolated them with a hemostat and tied them off. Five packs of suture later, all of the bleeders were under control. At 6:10 p.m., Allie released all the pressure from the tourniquet. We made it! She left it loose around Captain's elbow in case I dislodged a ligature while flushing the wound. At first, large pieces of road dirt dropped to the floor. By the third liter, no visible debris remained.

The clean wound now needed a wet-to-dry bandage for protection. I put on a fresh pair of gloves, and Allie dropped several sterile gauze pads into my hands. I placed them over the entire wound and dripped sterile fluid over them, forming the "wet" part of the bandage. Next, I covered the gauze with pads containing a waterproof barrier on the outer surface. All these layers were held in place by cast padding, roll gauze and a final layer of vet wrap. Only the tips of Captain's toes protruded from the bottom of the wrap by the time I finished. Bright red wrap covered the rest of his leg. I secured the end of the vet wrap with a piece of medical tape.

"Can I get Jennifer now?" Allie asked. She turned off the EKG machine and removed the leads, which left clamp marks in Captain's skin. When she removed the oxygen mask, Captain opened his eyes and yawned. He arched his back as he stretched his entire body. He even lifted his bandaged leg off the table!

"Let's clean this mess up first. Jennifer looked like she was going to pass out before," I replied. Blood, fur and debris covered the towel on the floor. I folded up the towel, trapping the dirt inside. With my gloves still in place, I picked it up and ran for the bathtub. A trail of bloody fluid followed my footsteps. Allie mopped up the mess. She surveyed the room one last time before leaving.

"Everything looks good so I'll go get her," Allie said as she turned to leave.

"Better clean off your arm first." I pointed at her right arm where a streak of blood extended from her elbow down her arm. She raised it to examine the bloodstain.

"Yikes!" She washed it off at the scrub sink. "See any other spots, Dr. Nelson?" She twirled in place.

"No, you look good." I looked at myself. "How about me?" I spun around.

"You're clothes look fine but you have quite a bit of splatter on your shoes." I looked down. Tiny spots of blood covered the tops. I moistened a paper towel with disinfectant and wiped the tops of my shoes.

When Jennifer entered the treatment room, Captain rolled from his side onto his chest. He knocked the folded towel off the table as he extended his legs. Jennifer ran to Captain's side, threw her arms around his neck and hugged him. The dog wagged his tail. When Jennifer relaxed her grip, he turned his head toward her, studying her face for a few seconds. His nose twitched from side to side, and his tail froze in place as he drank in Jennifer's scent. After three more sniffs, Captain leaned into Jennifer and licked her face.

Her eyes filled with tears, she buried her face in Captain's thick fur. "I'm so sorry," she whispered over and over again.

"As you can see, Jennifer, Captain is doing much better." I removed a box of tissues from the shelf above the treatment table and placed them on the table. "He's out of shock and feeling better after the pain medicine." Jennifer straightened up and blew her nose. "Now the big problem is the leg." I pointed at the thick bandage. It concealed a horrible injury.

"Is he going to lose it?" Jennifer asked with trepidation.

I shook my head and smiled. I explained that Captain could move his toes, which indicated the nerves to his paw were intact. His paw also felt warm to the touch, so the blood supply was still functioning. The biggest problem facing him now was infection. It wasn't a question of if the wound was infected but what it was infected with. Jennifer nodded and tried to comprehend despite her shock and emotion.

"For the next few days, we'll flush Captain's leg twice per day," I told her. "When the wound stops weeping, I'll evaluate it for closure." I warned her that the wound might require a skin graft.

"When can I bring him home?"

"Let's see, today is Friday." I thought for a moment. "The first three days are the worst for these kinds of injuries. Captain will need frequent bandage changes and lots of medicine to control his pain. If everything goes according to plan, you'll be able to take him home sometime next week."

"Blake is going to be so upset," Jennifer said, placing her hand on her forehead. "Captain sleeps in bed with him at night."

"Bring him in for a visit," Allie responded. "We're open on Saturday from 8 till noon."

"What do you mean, we're open?" I asked Allie. "Steve and I will be slaving away in the clinic while you're sleeping in."

"And what's wrong with that?" Allie winked at me and grinned.

"Seriously, Jennifer, we want people to visit their pets while they're in the hospital." I petted Captain's head. "It seems to make them feel better. They heal faster."

"Blake and I will be here tomorrow as soon as I pick him up from his father's house," Jennifer said. She took Captain's head in both of her hands and stared into his brown eyes. "Rest well, little teddy bear. I'll see you tomorrow." With that, Captain planted another sloppy kiss on his owner's chin.

CHAPTER 18

Emily the Guinea Pig

Overnight temperatures plummeted to the low teens. Slush froze into bizarre, uneven shapes. Hunks of gray ice littered the roads. Snowplows dumped their loads of salt and sand on icy patches. Sand accumulated in the center of traffic lanes. Most cars sported long black icicles behind each tire. If the driver made a sharp turn, the back edge of the tire ground into the icicle.

Steve and I parked as usual toward the highway and away from the building. We always left the close spaces open for clients. When I got out of the car, I noticed an especially long clump of ice stuck behind the tire well. I kicked it with the toe of my boot. Sharp pain radiated through my toes. The clump did not move.

A thin sheet of ice covered the surface of the parking lot. Steve slid his hand around my arm as we made our way to the front door. White pellets of salt lay on the building sidewalk. I took off a mitten and inserted a gold-colored key into the lock. My fingers tingled from the cold metal. The key refused to turn in the lock. I jiggled the door handle with my other hand and tried again.

"What's wrong?" Steve asked. The edges of his ears beneath his hat were bright pink.

"I think the lock is frozen." I dangled the keychain in front of him. "Do you want to give it a try?"

He pulled off his green leather gloves and tried it. "It's frozen stiff," he said. "I'm afraid to put too much pressure on the key; it might break off in the lock." He raised his hands up to his mouth and blew into them. "We need some lock deicer."

I opened the black nylon work bag that hung from my shoulder. The month before, one of our vendors had given me a purse-size lock deicer. Now if I could only find it among the scrubs, protein bars, toothbrush, toothpaste, brush, lip gloss and other junk. I pushed the contents from one side to the other.

"I'm afraid your bag is a like a black hole, dear," Steve observed. "Maybe we should ..."

"Found it." I pulled a little metal can out of a pocket, snapped a delivery straw into the nozzle and handed it to Steve. He sprayed two blasts into the lock and inserted the key again. The deadbolt slid back into the door.

"After you, my dear," Steve said as he held the door open for me. "I can't believe I married a woman who carries lock deicer in her purse."

"And kitty litter in her trunk," I added. "Just in case the Probe needs traction."

"You've come a long way from breaking off the shift handle of the old farm truck," he said with a smile.

By 8 a.m., Steve and I finished our morning duties. Captain sported a new fluorescent green bandage on his leg. The birds dined on fresh vegetables for breakfast. Genny nibbled on her cat food and then set out to explore the clinic. Every morning, she conducted "rounds." She rubbed her face on door-jambs, cabinets and walls to let the rest of the world know this was her clinic and drew wicked delight being outside the cages. This three-legged cat was the envy of the hospitalized patients locked behind bars.

Our first appointment was a hamster who chewed off his fur, a condition called barbering. The owner said his backside look liked the haircut their 3-year-old daughter gave the cat. Clumps of hair were missing here and there. I hoped this was a nice hamster – the last one I treated sunk her teeth into my thumb when I tried to pick her up.

For the next hour, the phone rang nonstop with cancellations. The first call came from the hamster's owner. Their car would not start. Another client slipped on the ice and was on the way to the emergency room with a broken wrist. An hour ticked by without any appointments. With each phone call, Steve became concerned. He was tired of helping each Saturday. But to hire another technician, I needed more revenue. I hated to burden him, but there was no other way.

At 9:30 a.m., our first visitor arrived, the mail lady. She wore thick wool pants tucked in heavy-duty boats, a thick winter jacket and suede mittens. A very unstylish blue-grey babushka perched on her head, the flaps covering her ears completely. It was not a look destined to appear in Vogue. When she entered the clinic, her glasses fogged over from the warmth, but she looked over the tops of them to survey my plants.

"The plants are looking much better," she observed.

"Yes, we followed your advice, and it made a big difference," I replied. "Thanks for the help." She smiled as the door opened behind her. In walked a woman with a chocolate Lab and a poodle dressed in a leather jacket. The black bomber jacket stood out against her curly white hair. The Lab bounded toward the mail lady with a silly grin on her face, sniffing the mailbag until her owner pulled her away.

"I'm glad you braved the weather to come and see us this morning," Steve said.

"Oh, it's not that bad if you dress for it," the woman replied. She removed her mittens, unbuttoned her coat and walked over to the counter. "We are the Davenports. I'm Stacy; that's Lady." She pointed to the lab. "And this is Cleopatra." She held the tiny poodle up to Steve.

"What are the girls here for today?" Steve asked.

"I found a lump on Cleo's breast that I want checked out. Lady is just here for moral support," she answered.

"Good for you, Lady," Steve responded. While Stacy filled out the information sheet, I watched Lady walk around the lobby. She threw her front legs out to the side in a big circle without bending her elbows. She also carried more weight than normal on her back legs.

"Does Lady have elbow dysplasia?" I asked.

Stacy nodded. "The condition was diagnosed when she was 6 months old. The vet told me to put her to sleep and get another dog." She reached down and patted Lady's head. "But I couldn't do that to Lady. She's part of the family."

"I'm glad you didn't listen. She can live a relatively pain-free life if you limit her exercise to low-impact activities and keep her weight down," I offered. Stacy nodded.

"And I give her lots of joint supplements as well," she continued. "I think she has a pretty good life." Lady closed her eyes and let her tongue fall out of her mouth as Stacy continued to pet her.

Steve escorted the Davenports to the dog room, but Lady spotted the aquarium in the cat room. She lunged toward the glass, pulling the leash out of Stacy's hand. A few inches from the tank, Lady screeched to a halt, mesmerized by the fish inside. Since Lady wanted to watch the fish, we accommodated her and moved into the cat room.

Cleopatra stood with all four legs perfectly aligned on the exam table as if she were at Madison Square Garden for Westminster. One by one, I checked each mammary gland. Mammary tumors come in all sizes and shapes. Aggressive carcinomas often break through the skin. Owners see blood, then notice the lump. A common benign tumor often occurs under the nipples and feels like a hard BB.

"What do you think, Dr. Nelson?" Stacy asked in a nervous voice.

Between my fingers, I held a firm mass. The edges felt irregular. The top felt pitted like a cobblestone street missing a stone here and there. Red streaks radiated out from the mass into the surrounding skin. Beside the first lump, I felt another smaller one. In dogs, 50 percent of mammary gland tumors are malignant. The odds are far worse in cats – breast tumors are almost always malignant.

"I'm afraid I found two lumps," I finally responded. Stacy's eyes widened. "Cleo needs to have them removed as soon as your schedule allows." I pointed to the bigger mass. "This one worries me." I have a duty to be honest with each client about the pet's medical condition. But I felt horrible giving this news to Stacy. "We'll send the lumps to the lab and it will take about a week to get a diagnosis from the pathologist. I'll also have them check the borders to see if I got clean margins during the surgery." Stacy held Cleo to her chest and stroked the little dog.

"But you really don't know what kind of cancer it is. I mean," her voice cracked, "it could be benign, right?" I nodded, but something told me not to be optimistic. Stacy kissed Cleo's forehead. Her eyes glistened with tears. Lady appeared by Stacy's side with her tail tucked between her legs. She knew something was wrong. We scheduled Cleo's surgery for Monday. Stacy put the leather jacket back on Cleo and left without saying a word.

"What's wrong with Cleo?" Steve asked as her van pulled away.

"She has two lumps in her breasts," I replied quietly. Steve stood in silence. Just saying those words cast a shadow over the clinic. We both hoped surgery would cure the little fashion plate.

"Anything good in the mail?" I asked, trying to change the subject. He shook his head and handed me a stack of envelopes.

"I keep forgetting to ask if you heard any more from the clinic that sent you the nasty letter," he said.

"No, I guess our attorney wrote a good poison-pen response." I smiled and thumbed through the mail. "So what's next on the books?"

"Nothing, except Ivan Harris is coming in at noon. Rich thinks
he has another hotspot, and it's time to recheck his thyroid level."
Steve spun around in the desk chair. "Jennifer and her son are in
back visiting Captain. Good job on the green. The bandage
matches the boy's mittens, scarf and hat – green is his favorite
color."

I winked at Steve. Steve's favorite color was also green. Besides
gloves, he had a green winter jacket, a green car and lots of green
ties for work. I, on the other hand, liked purple. My childhood bedroom was purple from top to bottom with purple carpeting, purple
drapes and vinyl jungle wallpaper in shades of purple, blue and
lemon yellow. It was extreme purple.

Ivan arrived at the clinic just as Jennifer and Blake finished
their visit. Blake clung to his mother when he saw the large
Doberman. Rich kept Ivan by his side. When the coast was clear,
he unclipped the leather leash from Ivan's silver choke collar,
which sparkled next to his black coat. Ivan sniffed the chairs Genny
had marked earlier in the day and started to lift his leg on one.

"Ivan, no," Rich ordered. The dog gave him a look that said,
"What? I wasn't going to do anything." Steve ushered Rich and
Ivan into the pharmacy area where there was more room to work
on the large dog. Ivan strutted in with his head held high. Lack of
confidence was not his problem.

"Hello, hello," Bongo called out. Ivan's head jerked toward the
mechanical voice. He trotted to her cage with Rich trailing behind
and stood like a statue in front of the cages. His eyes darted from
one bird to another.

"Hey, Dobermans aren't supposed to be bird dogs," I called out.
"Ivan, come." Ivan looked at me for a second, wagged his little
stump of a tail but failed to move his feet. He returned his attention
to the birds.

"Come on, boy," Rich said as he slid his hand under the collar.
"Sorry, Kris, sometimes he's such a butthead." Rich pulled Ivan to
me. He removed his leather jacket and tried to hang it on the office

doorknob, but for some reason, it kept falling to the floor. I took it from him, brushed off some dog fur and laid it over a chair in the office.

Ivan stood facing the birds for the entire exam. He didn't move a muscle unless I blocked his view. On the inner side of his back left leg, I found a quarter-sized area of moist pink skin. Rich noticed the spot in the morning and called right away. I gathered supplies from the cabinet and laid them on the floor next to Ivan.

"Ivan, platz," Rich ordered in German. Ivan looked at Rich but did not lie down. The owner stared at him with a look that said, "I'm not kidding," and with that, Ivan sank. With Rich's help, I treated the hotspot and drew blood from a small vein in Ivan's back leg.

"OK, we're done," I announced as I filled a test tube with bright red blood. Ivan sprang to his feet. He knew what OK meant. Rich grabbed his collar before he could run back to the birds and reattached the leash. "I'll call with the thyroid results on Monday," I told him.

While I was busy with Ivan, Genny noticed the strange jacket on the chair and came out of the closet to inspect. She stood below it, sniffing the hem. After several minutes, she jumped onto the chair and buried her face it. Rich had purchased the jacket in Italy during a recent business trip. Made of high-quality leather and soft as butter, the jacket emitted that wonderful new leather smell. Genny, however, was entranced by the tactile sensation. She pushed her paws into the jacket's folds, shifting her weight back and forth. Before long, she was lost in the world of forbidden pleasure.

I opened the door to find Genny holding the collar in her mouth, kneading the leather with her front paws and a glassy look on her face. When I picked her up and placed her on the floor, she protested with a loud "waa, waa." I picked up the jacket and inspected it for damage. "Rich, Genny was on your jacket. I'm really sorry about that. I didn't know she liked leather."

"Oh, that's alright," Rich replied. "She can sleep on it."

"That's not what she was doing. Genny was, ah, she was, ah, ah ... well, let's just say she loves your leather jacket." I raised my hands and wiggled the first two fingers on each hand in quotes as I uttered the word "loves." Rich looked at me quizzically. I paused for a moment as I searched for a nice way to say what Genny was doing. "She loves your jacket ... in a sexual way."

"You mean she did the wild thing on my jacket?"

I nodded. Rich started to chuckle, which grew to a full laugh. The more he thought about what Genny was doing, the harder he laughed. His face turned red.

Steve walked into the room, wondering what was taking so long. "We just got a walk-in, Kris, a guinea pig with an injured leg. The owners think it might be broken." Rich continued to laugh. He put on his jacket and coiled Ivan's leash in his hand. "Come on, Ivan, let's get out of here." Ivan reluctantly turned his attention from the birds and followed him out the door.

Earlier in the day, Jeff and Laurie Shultz had stopped by the local Humane Society with their children. They wanted to adopt a small pet that would be comfortable in their apartment. After looking at many animals, they selected a beautiful young guinea pig with a bright white coat and pink eyes. Their daughter, Maria, named the precious snowball Emily. On the way home, they stopped at a pet store and purchased the necessary accessories including food, litter, a bright pink harness and matching leash. Three hours later, Emily caught her back leg in the leash. She limped around after that without touching the injured foot to the ground.

I examined Emily just like every other pet, starting at her head and finishing with her injured right rear leg. The foot was normal, but just above the hock I noticed a swollen area. Emily jerked her leg back and tried to escape when I touched it. Further inspection revealed a puncture wound on the inner side of her leg.

"I'm worried that Emily has an open fracture," I announced to the family with the guinea pig perched in one hand. "See this hole in her skin?" I pointed to the puncture wound. "I'm worried that her bone popped through the skin when it broke. Infection is a big problem in wounds like this." Silence fell over the family. Tears rolled down the daughter's cheeks. She hid her face in her mother's coat.

X-rays confirmed what I already knew. Emily's fracture occurred through the growth plate of her tibia. Technically, it is called a Salter II fracture. The entire family followed me into the treatment room to view the film.

"Can you fix it?" Jeff asked.

I took a deep breath before answering. Fractures like this can be tough to repair for several reasons. First, the fracture went right through the growth plate. As the name suggests, it's the area where bone lengthens during growth. If the cells in that area were badly damaged, her leg would not grow properly. Second, guinea pig bones are like chicken bones, thin and fragile. I would have to be careful not to damage it further during surgery. Third, the bone was contaminated with bacteria and dirt. Infection was a big issue. To make matters worse, guinea pigs don't respond well to anesthesia. With her young age and small size, I warned the family that she might not make it through the anesthesia.

"But she needs the leg fixed, right?" Laurie stated. "I mean, she can't live with a broken leg."

"Yes," I answered. "I will put a wrap on the leg to stabilize the fracture. Once it stops moving, she will feel a lot better." I smiled at the girl, who was still upset. "The bandage will make it feel better just like when you put a bandage on an owie," I told her. I flipped off the light box. "I can fix the fracture on Monday."

"Dr. Nelson," Maria whispered. "Emily needs to be home for Easter. Take good care of her."

"I'll do my best," I replied.

After the family left, Steve held little Emily for me. I clipped the hair from her leg and flushed the wound with saline. Once the leg was dry, I applied a soft padded bandage. I cut a tongue depressor to the perfect size for her little leg and wrapped it into the bandage for support.

Emily felt a lot better with the leg stabilized. She hopped around the incubator, leaving a long noseprint along the glass. Her limp was slight. She ate a teaspoon of pellets, sipped a little water and settled into the corner for a nap.

"Poor little thing," I said as we stood observing her. "She's had quite a day."

"Yeah, but she got a good home with people who care," Steve replied. He took my hand in his. "I have a good feeling about Emily. I think she's going to do just fine. Let's follow her lead and get some lunch. I'm starving."

CHAPTER 19

Sugar and Spice, Maltese Sisters

Ben O'Brian returned home from a frustrating day at work. He opened the front door expecting a warm welcome from Sugar and Spice, his two Maltese. At 10, Sugar was the calm, friendly dog. When she stood, her legs bowed into abnormal positions. Her wrists caved forward onto her front paws while her hocks bent backwards almost to the ground. But what she lacked in physical beauty, she made up for in personality. She was Miss Congeniality with a capital C.

Spice lived up to her name. She zipped from place to place. Her motto was "Why walk when you can run?" The muscles on her body bulged beneath curly white fur. Because Ben rescued Spice from an abusive situation, she was shy and nervous around strangers. She let Sugar meet them first while she watched from the safety of Ben's arms.

Ben opened the door to an empty foyer. His voice echoed down the hall as he called for his girls. "Sugar, Spice, where are you?" Silence greeted him. Without removing his coat, he walked down the hallway in search of his dogs. Spice met him at the doorway to the kitchen. Instead of jumping into his arms for a hug, she touched his hand with her nose and ran toward the back of the house. Ben knew something was terribly wrong. Spice never left Sugar's side.

When he reached the bedroom, his concern became panic. Sugar lay on her side in the middle of the floor with her legs stretched outward. Her nostrils flared with each breath. Spice stood by her side and whimpered.

"Sugar," Ben cried. "What's wrong?" Sugar raised her head one inch off the ground. She looked at him for two seconds, moved her tail once and collapsed. Ben knelt beside her and put his hand on her chest. He felt it rise and fall with each breath. Sugar closed her eyes. It was as if she used her last bit of energy to greet Ben. She fought to stay alive long enough to say goodbye.

Snatching a blanket from the hall closet, Ben wrapped it around Sugar, grabbed his car keys and headed for the front door with the dog's limp body in his arms. "Hang on, Sugar," he whispered as tears spilled down his cheeks. "Please don't die." Spice followed, whining. She knew her friend was in serious trouble. When Ben got to the car, he could hear Spice howling as he laid Sugar on the front seat. Spice's cries sounded like the frantic wails of someone losing her best friend.

At the clinic, squealing brakes caused Allie to look up from her paperwork. Through the clinic window, she watched Ben slam his car into park in front of the clinic. He threw open the door, ran to the passenger side and scooped up his beloved pet. Allie ran to the front door and held it open.

"This is Sugar," Ben said as he walked inside. "I got home from work and found her on the floor." He spoke in staccato bursts. Allie pointed to the cat room with one arm and nudged Ben's elbow with the other.

"She was just laying there." Ben lowered his voice. "She ... she even peed on the floor." Allie flipped on the lights and motioned for Ben to place Sugar on the table. "That's not like her. She never would do that." Beads of sweat formed on his forehead. His fair skin flushed to a bright pink.

Allie lifted Sugar's lip and pressed on the gum above the big canine tooth. The color returned in a second, but her gums were slightly pale. Next, Allie took the stethoscope from her scrub pocket. She placed the bell of the instrument on Sugar's chest. Allie stood watching the second hand circle the Starship Enterprise for one minute as she counted Sugar's heart rate. Ben stood close to his dog, watching every move Allie made. Finally, she stuck a thermometer in Sugar's rear end. Sugar did not resist; she just lay there and panted.

"101.8," she said smiling. Ben's facial expression did not change. "That's normal for a dog." She opened Sugar's record and recorded her findings on a new physical exam sheet. "Dr. Nelson will be in right away." She patted Sugar's head and left.

When I entered the room, Ben was sitting next to Sugar with his arm across her back. He positioned the exam room chair tight to the exam table. His gray-white hair matched Sugar's snowy white coat. They looked like a match made in heaven.

Ben cuddled his pet as he recounted the events of the day. Nothing was out of the ordinary when he left for work. Sugar and Spice got a biscuit and went to their beds as usual. He hadn't changed their diets. No exposure to any kind of poison. Ben kept all the chemicals he used for cleaning in a locked cabinet. She was not on any kind of medication and did not have any drug allergies as far as he knew.

"Any coughing, sneezing, vomiting or diarrhea?" I asked. Ben shook his head no. I closed the cover of Sugar's record. "Well, let's take a look at you, pumpkin." Sugar looked up at me and tried to jump off the table. When that failed, she tried to jump into Ben's arms. I performed the physical exam with her sitting in Ben's lap. Other than her bowed legs and slightly pale gums, I couldn't find anything to explain what happened.

Fortunately, her breathing had improved dramatically since arriving at the clinic. I suspected that Sugar suffered a seizure but was unsure of the cause. I sent blood and urine off to the lab for tests. Ben took Sugar home while we waited for the results. He placed my pager number in his wallet just in case Sugar had problems during the night.

The next day Ben brought Sugar back for observation while he was at work. Her condition had deteriorated overnight. When I called her name, she thumped her tail a few times but kept her head on the table. Her gums were now a faint pink. I pulled the stethoscope from around my neck and positioned the bell over her chest. "Whoosh, whoosh, whoosh" echoed in my ears. I feared Sugar had autoimmune hemolytic anemia – a lack of red blood cells causing her murmur.

I held Sugar as Allie drew blood. We mixed one drop with saline and placed the rest in a purple-top tube. The red bloods cells clumped into pieces the size of pepper.

"Her blood just agglutinated," I said holding up the slide for Allie to view.

"It's clumped in here, too." Allie inverted the blood tube in her hand. Clumps of cells floated from one side to the other like an inverted snow globe. "I've never seen one this bad."

As Allie helped me place an IV catheter in Sugar's malformed leg, I thought about the other dogs I had treated with this condition. Autoimmune hemolytic anemia is a life-threatening disease. The patient makes antibodies against its own red blood cells. The antibodies attach to these cells and signal the spleen to discard them. It destroys the red blood cells, causing a life-threatening anemia. If the process is not stopped, the patient will die. We had to end this process now to save Sugar. The textbooks in my office made it sound so easy. Combine massive doses of steroids with good nursing care, and the patient recovers. In practice, I learned that textbooks seldom tell the whole story.

The test results from the prior day showed a slightly low packed-cell volume (PCV) and some problems with the morphology of the red blood cells. Specifically, the pathologist observed cells shaped like little targets, a tell-tale sign of autoimmune disease. Her PCV dropped to 18 percent on the sample we analyzed this morning. If it dropped much further, she would need a blood transfusion. Although donor red blood cells would carry oxygen throughout Sugar's body, they also would contain antigens foreign to Sugar's immune system. Even with a cross-match, the donor red blood cells would make it more difficult to get her under control with steroids. I administered large doses of steroids and hoped to keep her PCV out of the critical range.

The sun shone brightly as Ben drove to the clinic after work. Areas of dormant grass appeared between piles of dirty snow. Green buds lined barren tree branches. After months of cold and snow, the promise of spring was in the air, but Ben was oblivious. He thought only of Sugar. What would he do if she didn't make it? He tried to push those thoughts out of his mind.

Allie escorted him to the treatment room as soon as he arrived. In the pharmacy, he noticed Genny in front of the refrigerator. She stood on her one back leg and tried to reach a homemade card with her front paws. Two magnets kept it firmly out of reach. A hand-drawn guinea pig adorned the cover with "Emily" scribbled below. Inside, a stick-figure family shouted "Thank you."

"Who's this little fellow?" Ben asked.

"That's Genny, our clinic cat. Dr. Nelson rescued her last summer," Allie said as Genny gave up on the card and sat down.

Ben stopped for a better look. "What happened to her leg?"

"We're not really sure," Allie explained. "The foot was missing when Dr. Nelson adopted her."

"Poor little thing," Ben said in amazement. Genny sauntered over to Ben and sniffed his pants and shoes. Ben bent down and scratched the little tortoiseshell under the chin. She let out an annoyed meow and swatted his hand with her front paw. Ben jumped back, shocked by her behavior. He clearly was uninitiated in the ways of Genny.

"She's pretty spoiled," Allie commented. "Everything has to be on her terms or else."

"Sounds like some of the people I work with," Ben replied.

Sugar rested in one of the middle cages, about waist high off the ground. She lay on her chest like a sphinx, her head resting on a rolled-up towel across her front legs. This position made it easier for her to breathe. A bag of Lactated Ringer's solution hung on the front of her cage with the clear fluid dripping into the attached line at a slow rate.

Ben winced at the sight of his beloved pet. "Sugar, Sugar," he whispered. She opened her eyes, and her tail moved back and forth slowly. Allie opened the cage door and rearranged the I.V. line. Ben froze in place about two feet from the cage, not sure what to do next. Allie motioned for him to come closer. He moved forward two steps and placed his hand on Sugar's head. She licked it with her pale pink tongue. Ben swallowed hard, his eyes glistening with tears. He reached into the cage and cuddled his dog's head with both of his hands. Sugar closed her eyes again, her chest continuing to heave with every breath. She used most of her energy for breathing.

Allie walked into the office. I looked at her with the phone pressed between my shoulder and ear. "Yes, Stacy Davenport, please, may I speak to Stacy Davenport? This is Dr. Nelson calling with lab results." Allie pulled a piece of scrap paper from her pocket and scribbled a note. She laid it on the desk. I heard a loud click on the phone and the elevator music ended.

"Hello, this is Stacy," a female voice said.

"Stacy, I've got great news for you," I blurted into the phone. "Cleopatra's lumps are benign."

"Benign," she repeated.

"That's right Stacy," I paused. "And the margins are clean." Silence filled the space between us. After all of Stacy's sleepless nights, it seemed surreal.

"That's wonderful," she finally answered. Her voice quivered as spoke. "I was so worried."

"Me too," I echoed. "But it was benign, so now I want you to check her once a week for lumps. Other than that, you are under strict orders to spoil her rotten."

"I can do that," Stacy replied with joy. "I can definitely do that."

I hung up the phone, still filled with elation over the news. Sometimes misdiagnosing is wonderful. I stood up and headed back to the treatment room. Ben remained in the same position with Sugar's head in his hands. I stood by his side in silence, not wanting to interrupt the moment of pure love.

"She doesn't look too good," Ben said without looking at me. "Is she going to make it?" Tears streamed down his face.

"Her PCV continues to drop. It was 29 percent yesterday, 18 percent this morning and 16 percent at the last check." I moved closer to Ben. The orange cat in the next cage stuck his paw through the bars and meowed. "I'm hoping the steroids will kick in soon so she can avoid a blood transfusion."

"She's breathing so hard," Ben whispered. "She barely wagged her tail to greet me."

"That's because she's trying to conserve oxygen," I replied. She has about one-fourth her normal blood capacity to carry oxygen." I managed a small smile. "She's doing exactly what she should be."

Ben nodded his head and continued to stroke her head. "Do you think seeing Spice might perk her up?" For the first time, he looked at me with a glimmer of hope shining in his eyes. "I would be happy to run home and get her."

"I don't think she's ready for that yet." Ben looked down at Sugar again, deflated. "But that's a great idea for when she's better. I think it would do her and Spice a world of good." The glimmer evaporated from Ben. He kissed Sugar and wiped the tears from his cheeks before leaving. I know Ben wondered if he would ever see his old girl alive again.

By 10:30 that night, Sugar's PCV fell to 10 percent. The massive doses of steroids had failed to stop the disease. Her spleen continued to destroy the few remaining red blood cells. Sugar needed a blood transfusion, and she needed it now. Where was I going to find a donor at this hour? Steve and I thought through our family and friends. My sister was always a good sport about helping me out, even in the middle of the night. Unfortunately, her shit tsu, Tai Paws, tipped the scale at a whopping 14 pounds. Sugar needed more blood than Tai Paws could safely donate.

"How about one of the Harris dogs?" Steve suggested. One by one, I ticked off their pets in my mind. Ivan has too many health issues. I wouldn't want to stress his immune system. Bonnie and Clyde are too old, but Lulu ... she would be perfect. Now I just had to convince them to bring her in.

Linda and her husband, Rich, love animals. When Linda was young, she used to carry turtles across the road to keep them safe. Rich rescued their Saint Bernard, Lulu, from a horrific situation. The kennel used her as a bait dog to train pit bulls to fight. They taped her mouth closed and then let the puppies attack her. The tips of her ears were shredded and frayed from the abuse she suffered.

"Hello, Harris residence," Linda answered. I could hear the TV in the background.

"Hi, Linda, I'm sorry to call so late, but I need your help," I said. "I've got a sick dog at the clinic that needs a transfusion. I was wondering if I could draw some blood from Lulu?" Linda agreed without hesitation.

Rich arrived at the clinic with Lulu 15 minutes later. I cross-matched a small sample of her blood with Sugar's. Lulu nosed around the clinic chasing a syringe case, a Scruffy leftover. I gave her a mild tranquilizer and placed an I.V. catheter in her front leg. While I drew blood from Lulu's neck, clear fluid dripped into her veins to keep her blood pressure up. She passed the time watching Genny play with Rich's shoelaces. I locked his leather jacket in a safe place.

Forty-five minutes later, Lulu's blood dripped into Sugar's veins. With each burgundy drop, Sugar's condition improved. Her breathing became less labored, and a faint pink color returned to her gums. When half the bag was gone, Steve laid out two sleeping bags on the floor and put Genny back in her room. She meowed and stuck her paw under the door. We took turns throughout the night napping and watching Sugar.

The next day, when Ben arrived for his afternoon visit, Sugar looked much better. Her gums were pink, her respirations normal and her murmur was gone.

The clinic buzzed with animals and people. Spring meant heartworm season in Minnesota. Dogs need an annual heartworm test and preventative for summer. In addition, the animals that had undergone surgery in the morning were ready to go home.

Instead of having Ben sit in the treatment room, Allie decided to bring Sugar up to the reception area. She capped off her fluid line and covered it with a pink bandage. Sugar wagged her tail every time Allie talked to her.

"Now it's time to go see Daddy." Sugar's tail thumped again.

Ben jumped to his feet when he saw his beloved pet in Allie's arms. Sugar squirmed and tried to get away from her. She wanted her Daddy. Allie directed Ben back into a chair and placed her on his lap. He wrapped his arms around her in a loving embrace. She snuggled into his side and licked him. She stared into his eyes as if memorizing his face. She adored him, and he adored her right back.

In between appointments, I headed up front to check on Sugar. She looked so happy in his lap. "Hi, Ben," I said, taking the seat next to him. "Doesn't she look good?" I patted her on the head.

"Yes, she has more energy today." He hugged her again. "That was awfully nice of those people to donate their dog's blood. Please thank them for me." I nodded. "Spice really misses Sugar. Last night she wouldn't get in bed with me. She paced around the house, looking for her buddy." Ben looked into Sugar's eyes. "Yes, Spice misses you, old girl."

"Bring her with you tomorrow," I replied. "I think it would be good for both of them." We chatted about the next 24 hours of Sugar's care. The transfusion had raised Sugar's PCV to 30 percent.

We would check her PCV twice a day. As soon as it stabilized, the dog could go home.

Sugar raised her head with an expectant look on her face when she heard her name. We both gazed at her and chuckled. "You are too smart, Miss Sugar," I said, patting her head. The expectant look disappeared. I stood to leave.

"Just one last thing before you go, Dr. Nelson." Ben cleared his throat before he continued. "I want you to call no matter what time of day or night if you think she's going to ..." He paused. "If you think she's going to..." Tears welled up in his eyes.

I placed my hand on his shoulder. "You will be the first to know if her condition changes. But hang in there, Ben. My money's on Sugar." Ben forced a smile in response. I only hoped I was right.

CHAPTER 20

Butch Revisited

Butch the Great Dane arrived with the entire family for his last set of puppy shots. Dan Arnold's wife, Joy, was a petite woman with sandy brown hair. She stood next to her husband, looking anxiously around the exam room. Butch sat at their feet listening to the activity in the waiting room. His head almost reached Dan's waist. The dog cocked his head back and forth, raising his ears occasionally.

A boy sat on a chair, his feet dangling. With his blond hair and blue eyes, he looked like a poster child for a Minnesotan of Scandinavian descent. He took off his jacket, placed it over his legs and kicked it for fun until Joy stopped him.

Dan interrupted me as I tried to introduce myself to his wife and son. He told me to make this quick as he needed to get home right away. Joy smiled briefly at me and mumbled hello before introducing her son, Dan Jr. I leaned over the exam table and stretched my arm out to the child.

"Can we get on with this?" Dan asked impatiently. As the child extended his hand toward me, I noticed scratches covered his arm. On closer inspection, I noted two deep puncture wounds. "He likes to play hard with Butch," Dan answered before I could ask. He hoisted Butch onto the table. "Whew, I think this will be his last time on the table."

During the last month, Butch's body transformed itself from pudgy puppy to awkward teenager. The parts of his body grew at different rates, making him look like he was comprised of spare parts from another animal. His broad head with its massive lips reminded me of the manatees I saw in Florida. His paws looked like they should be on a wolf. What impressed me the most was the growth of his torso. It was almost as long as my table. This pup was going to be a huge dog, even for a Great Dane.

Butch squirmed when I inserted the otoscope in his ear. "Would you mind putting a hand on him?" I asked Dan. He motioned for his wife to do it. She shuffled toward the table and gingerly placed her hands on the pup's neck. When I lifted his ear, he continued to squirm.

"Butch, no," she commanded with as stern a voice as she could muster. Butch ignored her. "Honey, he won't listen to me. Would you please hold him?" Dan smirked and rolled his eyes before exchanging places with his wife.

With Dan's assistance, I completed the rest of the exam in record time. Butch stood like a statue for his vaccinations. The pup stared at me after I completed the shots, but didn't make a sound. Due to my earlier work, he considered me superior, at least for now. Dan clipped a leather leash onto the ring of his collar and handed the other end to his wife. He grunted as he placed Butch on the ground.

"Take him to the car while I pay." Joy obediently opened the door, ushered Dan Jr. through it and started out. But Butch remained at Dan's feet. She pulled on the leash. Butch ignored her and continued to sit by Dan. "Butch, come!" she commanded. She walked over to the pup and attempted to raise his rear end off the ground. A low growl rumbled from his throat. She jerked her hands away from him. "Honey, will you take him?" she pleaded. Butch looked up at Dan and stopped growling. His ears perked and his tail waved back and forth.

"You go with her," he responded. Butch stopped wagging his tail and slowly followed Joy out of the room.

I thought for a moment before addressing Dan. How could I make him understand what was happening? I must choose my words carefully. "Dan, it looks like Butch will only obey you." I pulled a manila folder from the drawer. "I'm also concerned about the marks on your son's arms. Butch should never, ever be allowed to bite a human." Dan ignored me as he pulled his wallet from his pocket. "Even in play, it's too dangerous to let a big dog like Butch bite." Dan stared at me blankly. "Are you taking him to obedience classes?" He stood silently with his hands on his hips and turned toward the door without answering.

"Listen, Dan," I tried desperately to get his attention. "I'm concerned that Butch is an alpha dog. That means he wants to be the leader of the pack." He froze in his tracks.

"That's want I want." Dan turned toward me with a smile on his face. "Don't want no wusses at my house."

"But you don't understand," I continued undaunted. "Butch considers your family his pack. When he gets bigger, he will challenge you for that role. You need to get control of him now before it's too late and he hurts someone." Dan turned away from me again.

"See you in a year," he said as he left the room.

Back in the treatment room, Captain Thomas waited with Jennifer by his side. Blake stood in front of the cages, looking at the animals. A black cat rubbed back and forth on the bars in front of him. He scratched the cat's neck through the bars. Sugar slept in the cage next to him, snoring loudly, much to Blake's delight.

With school out for spring break, Jennifer took the week off of work. They planned a trip to The Minnesota Zoo when we finished the bandage change. I collected bandages from under the counter and retrieved a new box of vet wrap from the closet. "Blake, would you like to pick the color?" I opened the lid and bent over to show the variety of colors to the little boy. He pulled on his ear with one hand while pointing to a yellow roll with the other.

"You want yellow? I thought green was your favorite color," I said, pulling out the yellow roll and placing it next to the other bandages.

"Yellow is Grandma's favorite color," Blake replied.

"My Mom is coming to visit today," Jennifer explained. She tried to smooth the unruly hair on Captain's back. Allie usually held Captain for the bandage change because blood makes Jennifer queasy, but today Jennifer wanted to hold him. She promised to keep her eyes on me instead of Captain's wound.

I put Captain on the table and pushed his front legs out in front of him until his elbows rested on the table. Jennifer and I rolled him onto his left side. Captain squirmed, then quieted. Holding still was tough for him. I inserted the tips of a heavy-duty bandage scissors into the wrap over Captain's toes. The blades cut through the layers of padding one small bite at a time. By the time I reached the top, the handles left impression marks over my knuckles.

"OK, I'm going to take the bandage off. Don't look," I said. Jennifer turned her head away. "How in the world did you manage to get him in here after the accident with all that blood? I am amazed you did not pass out."

"I almost did after I got to the clinic. All that blood," she shrugged her shoulders. "I kept thinking about Captain."

I peeled the bandage off from top to bottom, following the direction of hair growth. Captain cried when I pulled the tape stirrups off his skin. The wound had made remarkable progress since the accident; it was about half its original size, and healthy pink granulation tissue covered the bone and tendons.

I explained my observations to Jennifer. Since the bone was covered, she felt she could look at the wound without passing out. She turned her head for a quick peek. Her face flashed white, and she swallowed hard. My own stomach jumped to my throat. I am comfortable with sick animals, but sick people are another story.

Jennifer leaned forward and cleared her throat. When she straightened up, her color was back to normal. I would never trust her near open wounds again.

Now that granulation tissue covered the wound, Jennifer had a decision to make. At this stage we could continue to bandage the wound and let it heal on its own, or it could be covered with a skin graft. The graft would speed up healing time, but it required putting Captain under anesthesia, something that made Jennifer uncomfortable. The final cost of each would be about the same.

"I'd rather keep bandaging the leg," Jennifer replied without hesitation. "Now that we only have to come every other day, it's not so bad."

"Actually, I think we can go to every third day now. The wound isn't oozing much anymore."

"Fantastic!" Jennifer exclaimed. She bent down and rubbed her face in Captain's fur. After flushing the wound with saline, I covered it with a non-stick pad and applied a thick layer of cotton cast padding followed by stretch gauze. Per Blake's selection, bright yellow vet wrap topped it all off. I ripped a small piece of medical tape from the roll and used it to hold the end of the vet wrap in place. I wrote the date on the tape with a black marker.

"OK, you're all set." Captain sprang to his feet. He knew the word OK meant treat time. He watched me get a dog biscuit out of the jar. Just as Pavlov commanded, a drop of saliva dripped onto the table, and the pup's tail beat back and forth. I handed Captain the biscuit. When he finished, I hugged him for a long time relishing the moment. Eventually, I placed him gently on the floor. Standing up, I realized I was coated with fur, Captain's fur. It made me smile.

"I'll see you in three days," I said. Jennifer beamed with delight. For the first time since the accident, she knew in her heart that Captain would be all right. She had a twinkle in her eye, finally free of worry and guilt.

CHAPTER 21

Rusty the Blood Donor

O ver the next two days, Sugar's PCV declined again. Her body destroyed her own red blood cells and Lulu's too. She stopped eating. She seemed to be unaware of the animals and activities around her. The act of breathing exhausted her. She needed another transfusion.

Ben and Spice entered the clinic at their normal time to visit Sugar. Instead of her custom of bringing Sugar out to the waiting room, Allie ushered them to an exam room. As I entered, Ben sat on a chair in the corner with Spice on his lap. He clung tight to Spice and looked at me with a drawn, hollow face. His eyes were red. Sadness and concern hung over him; he knew the news was bad and was bracing for the worst.

"I'm afraid Sugar's PCV fell into the critical range again," I told him. I placed my hand on his arm. "She needs another transfusion." Ben leaned back in the chair, all hope and optimism draining from his body. The strong drugs I used were no match for Sugar's immune system. Her spleen destroyed the red blood cells faster than her body could make them. Her only hope was to remove her spleen to stop the destruction. I planned to give her another transfusion, then let her rest awhile before performing surgery.

Ben stared at the floor. Spice glanced at me for a second, then licked his face. "Do you think she can handle surgery?" he whispered.

"Not in her current condition," I paused. "But after a transfusion ... yes." I stepped back and waited for Ben to respond. Dark circles lined his eyes. Like Sugar, he looked exhausted.

He hugged Spice. "I ... I want to do whatever it takes to save her."

"That's the right decision, Ben." I opened the door. "All right, I'm going to make arrangements for the transfusion. Allie will get you in a minute. She's busy preparing for surgery on a dog that ate a bolt. Hang in there for me ... promise?"

I had met Rusty, the golden retriever, and Melanie Baylor last fall for a second opinion. Rusty experienced episodes of vomiting that worsened with time. Their veterinarian took X-rays but didn't see a problem. The films were "within normal limits," as radiologists like to say. The veterinarian sent Rusty home on conservative medical therapy. Unfortunately, the dog continued to vomit. Over the next 24 hours, the vomitus included blood. Melanie brought him back for more care, but once again, the vet could find no cause. After the third unsuccessful visit, the owner decided to try a new veterinarian. She brought Rusty to us, desperate for a cure.

During the exam, Rusty bounced off the walls. The young golden retriever had energy to burn. I agreed with my colleague; Rusty did not look sick. But Melanie said he was. Somewhere in my medical upbringing, I learned to listen to owners. They truly know what's normal for their pets.

During the first week of my internship at the Animal Medical Center in New York City, I examined a cat for lethargy. The owner said at home he barely moved. Yet the cat rubbed and purred throughout my examination. I thought he was the picture of health, but his owner insisted that something was wrong. I offered to perform blood tests and a urinalysis just to be sure. Lo and behold, the cat suffered from diabetes. From that moment on, I adhere to a healthy respect for owner intuition.

In young dogs, especially hunting dogs, the most common cause of vomiting is dietary indiscretion. That is a fancy term for eating the wrong thing. Unfortunately, not all foreign bodies show up on regular X-rays. I offered to perform a barium series to diagnose cloth and other non-mineral items. When the series was done, the diagnosis was easy. Rusty had a foreign body. I surgically removed about a foot of quilt batting from his small intestine.

Now, six months after the first surgery, Melanie brought Rusty in with the same symptoms. Again, he bounced off the walls during my examination. Allie and I struggled to hold him still for the X-rays. This time, the plain films made the diagnosis. Rusty had eaten a bolt, a big one with a washer attached.

As I changed into a set of scrubs, an idea popped into my head. Maybe I could use Rusty as a blood donor. His medical costs put a strain on his family's budget, and I could give them a credit for a blood donation. I grabbed Rusty's chart and headed for the phone.

"Hello, Baylor residence," a woman answered.

"Hi, Melanie, I'm calling to ask for your permission to use Rusty as a blood donor. I have a sick little Maltese here that desperately needs blood. If Rusty donates, I will credit your account for the donation."

"His eating habits have cost us a small fortune," she replied. She thought for a moment. "As long as it's safe for Rusty, I'm all for it."

"I won't draw from him until he's recovered from anesthesia and I know his blood is a match."

"Could you put a zipper in him, just in case he does this again?" Melanie asked, part in jest and part in earnest.

"Tempting, but not recommended." We both laughed.

"Someone must have done it, though," I said. "Some of the zipper packets actually state, 'Not for internal use.'" We laughed again.

Fifteen minutes later, I finished the surgical scrub and stood before the operating table dressed in cap, mask, gown and gloves. Rusty lay on his back with all four feet secured to the table with cords. Surgical instruments sat on a Mayo stand. I placed a series of small drapes on the dog's abdomen, leaving the center section open. Next, I covered his entire body with a blue paper drape. Allie sat by his head. As she reached under the drape to get his vitals, the EKG beeped in regular rhythm. I cut a hole in the drape to expose Rusty's abdomen.

The first surgery had left him with a long thin scar right down the middle. I followed the line with the scalpel blade. First skin, then subcutaneous tissues until the linea alba glistened under the bright O.R. lights. I punctured through with the tip of the scalpel, creating a hole big enough for my finger. I slid one inside for a quick feel. Because Rusty had surgery before, I had to be careful of adhesion between the incision and an internal organ. Feeling none, I methodically extended the incision with a scissors, using my finger to protect the vital organs below.

As surgeons, the natural tendency is to go directly to the problem and address it. In veterinary school, the instructors drilled into our heads the need to perform a thorough examination of the entire abdomen before undertaking anything else. I started at the diaphragm, reaching deep into Rusty's abdomen to feel its smooth surface. I slowly worked my way back past the spleen, kidneys and urinary bladder and finished by running the entire bowel from the stomach to the descending colon. The bolt in the stomach was the only abnormality.

Using lap sponges to isolate the stomach from the rest of the abdomen, I attached two pieces of suture to the outer wall and used them to pull the stomach up and out of the abdomen. I stabbed the area between the stay sutures with the scalpel blade. Blood oozed from the incision. I wiped it away before enlarging the incision with a scissors. Through the two-inch opening, I saw the bolt resting in the folds of the stomach. It had done a number on the stomach: the lining bled in places from denuded areas. I inserted a forceps through the incision and grabbed the bolt. I checked one more time for additional foreign bodies, then closed with a double layer of suture.

I changed into fresh gloves and got a new sterile set of instruments to avoid contaminating Rusty's abdomen. I removed the lap sponges and flushed the area with two liters of saline. The suction pump sputtered and squeaked as it vacuumed the fluid. Blood-tinged, it accumulated in the glass jar attached to the pump. I closed the abdominal incision one layer at a time. I knew from experience that Rusty would gnaw anything in his skin with his mouth. So this lucky dog was treated to the time-honored plastic surgeon closure. I buried the suture within the dermis, out of his reach.

Rusty shivered on the table as I pulled the drapes away. We moved him onto a thick quilt on the floor with a tracheal tube protruding from his mouth. Allie sat next to him, her hand on his back leg. She looked at her watch, counted his pulse and gently tapped the corner of his eyelid with a finger. When he blinked and coughed, she pulled out the trach tube. Rusty lifted his head and flicked his tongue from side to side.

An hour later, the dog stood in his run, ready to be a hero with his tongue hanging happily out the side of his mouth. His eyes sparkled with excitement. I could hear him barking from my office. Allie poked her head in the door.

"Hear that?" she asked.

"Is that who I think it is?"

"Yes. He's standing back there begging for dinner." Allie rolled her eyes. "I wish I had his energy."

"Me too." I smiled. "Let me give him a quick physical, and then he's all yours." I stood and stretched my arms. "And no food until tomorrow morning."

The next morning, I could hear Rusty's stomach rumble when

I listened to his chest. He jumped up and down in the run while I prepared a small meal for him. I opened his door just enough to slide the stainless steel bowl inside. He grabbed all the food in his mouth and swallowed it with one loud gulp. Standing on his back legs with his front feet resting on the wire gate, he looked at me with a grin on his face and wagged his tail.

"Woof, woof." The bark came from deep within.

"Nice try, Rusty." I reached over the gate to pet his head. "Begging won't work with me. Remember, I'm the mean old vet."

"Woof, woof," he barked again, wagging his tail so hard his entire body swayed from side to side. I smiled. I smiled big. It's hard to resist the charms of a happy dog.

Meanwhile, Sugar looked like a new dog with Rusty's blood coursing through her veins. The blood carried much-needed oxygen throughout her little body. She ate breakfast and for the first time in two days, walked outside under her own power. She looked great.

At noon, Rusty went home on a strict diet and medication to help his stomach ulcers. The top item on the go-home sheet instructed Melanie to get a basket muzzle for the dog. While Rusty could drink through the wire or plastic mesh, he could not eat anything.

At 3:30 p.m., Ben and Spice arrived for their daily visit. Ben sat in the same lobby chair with Sugar in his lap while Spice pranced on the floor, winding her leash around his legs. When she ran out of room, she stood on her back legs with her paws on Ben's knee. "Wrrrr, wrrr," she whined.

"What's wrong, Spice?" Ben cooed. "Did you tie yourself up in knots?" He unhooked the leash, picked her up and placed her next to Sugar. They watched other animals come and go from the safety of Ben's lap.

"Hi, Ben." I extended my right hand. "What do you think of her today?"

"She seems much better," he replied. He patted Sugar on the

head. "Maybe she won't need the splenectomy."

"It's possible," I said. I took a seat next to him. "It will depend on what her PCV is tomorrow morning. If it stays the same, she doesn't need surgery. If it drops, surgery is at 11 a.m."

"How is the dog who donated the blood? Is he OK?"

"Rusty is great. He didn't miss that blood at all. He went home at noon." I sat back into the chair with both hands on the armrests. My legs ached from walking the hard floors all day. "Rusty is a hyper dog. Sugar should be chasing Spice around in no time." Ben laughed at the thought with a zest he had not exhibited for some time.

"What do you think, Spice?" She looked into his eyes upon hearing her name. She had been watching a miniature pincher on the other side of the room. The small black-and-tan dog lay in his owner's lap with his ears perked up, looking like a regal sphinx. "Would you like it if Sugar chased you?" Spice put her paws on Ben's shoulder and licked his chin. "I think that's a yes."

"Well, I better get back to work," I said. "I've got a stack of medical records to finish." I stood and patted Sugar on the head. I extended my hand toward Spice, who leaned into Ben and hid her face in his jacket.

"Still shy after all this time," I said, shaking my head as I walked over to the counter for a medical record. "I'll call you tomorrow morning with the PCV. Keep your fingers crossed. Maybe we'll get lucky and she won't need surgery after all."

CHAPTER 22

Sugar's PCV Falls

Morning arrived with a cold drizzle. Sugar's body shivered against the chill as I took her outside. Her morning PCV fell six points from the day before. Ben was terrified at the thought of anesthesia, but he also knew it was Sugar's only hope. Reluctantly, he consented to a splenectomy.

"Dr. Nelson, will you do a favor for me?" he asked before we hung up.

"Certainly," I said.

"Tell her I love her." He paused and sniffled. "Tell her to hang on, and we'll be there to visit as soon as she's ready."

Allie set up the operating room while I saw the last appointment of the morning. She placed the water heating pad on the table, covered it with two towels and positioned the EKG machine at the head of the table. The cords wound around themselves into one big knot. She carefully detangled them according to color – green and white on one side and red and black on the other.

A splenectomy requires many forceps to clamp off blood vessels. Allie opened the surgical instrument cabinet. Blue and green packs of instruments closed by a piece of tape with black stripes lined the shelves. The tape looked like normal masking tape before it was autoclaved. Allie shifted around a few packs labeled "small" or "large spay" until she spotted a big one in the corner. From the size and weight, she knew it was the general surgery pack. She placed it on the Mayo stand along with sponges, suction equipment, drapes and a scalpel blade.

"Are you ready?" I asked when she returned to the treatment room. Allie handed me a cap and mask and nodded. She picked up Sugar and put her on the treatment room table. I picked up a syringe filled with clear liquid.

"Are you ready, Sugar?" I patted her head. She glanced up at me and licked her lips. I removed the cap and inserted the needle into a rubber catheter plug. Allie shut off the fluids to prevent back-flow. "Ben loves you, Sugar." Sugar blinked her eyes a couple times, opened her mouth in a wide yawn and then sank into Allie's arms.

Repositioning the dog on the table, Allie held Sugar's mouth wide open with both hands. I grabbed the dog's tongue with a piece of gauze, pulled it forward and waited for her to take a breath. On inhalation, I pushed the tip of a tracheal tube down her airway. Sugar sputtered and coughed. Allie connected the tube to the anesthesia machine, turned a valve for oxygen and flipped another switch for the isoflurane. The black bag attached to the machine moved with each of Sugar's breaths. After three more inhalations, the sputtering stopped.

"How's she doing?" I asked. Allie and I had worked together for over a year. I trusted her, something vital in the O.R. Allie held up her thumb as she listened with the stethoscope. Sugar's pulses were strong, and she breathed on her own. I gathered her limp body into my arms and carried her to the O.R., her head bouncing with every step I took. Allie followed with the anesthesia machine and I.V. pole.

Ten minutes later, I backed through the O.R. The EKG beeped in a regular, almost hypnotic, rhythm. Sugar rested on her back with a multitude of cords attached to her; her pink skin glistened under the bright O.R. lights.

Allie placed a headlamp on my head and tightened the head-band. She tied the cord into the back of my gown to keep it out of the way. I placed drapes on Sugar in much less time than it took for Rusty – girls are easier to drape. Next, I incised her skin one layer at a time until the internal organs sparkled under the head-lamp.

"Wow, look at the size of the spleen," I remarked. Allie stood on her tiptoes to get a peek. She kept her hands behind her back to avoid the sterile field.

"It's enormous," she said from under her mask. "It looks like the spleen that ate Minneapolis."

In dogs, the spleen is a narrow, flat organ that rests behind the stomach. It usually feels like a meaty sponge because of the many blood vessels that course through it. Sugar's spleen was thick and rounded, so much so that I found it difficult to perform the exploratory. Her huge spleen kept getting in the way.

I pulled the spleen out through the abdominal incision and laid it on the drapes. Allie opened a sterile package of lap sponges and dropped them on the Mayo stand, careful not to touch the sponges or contaminate the stand. I covered the spleen with the pads. Next, I poured saline over them to keep it moist.

Performing a splenectomy is a time-consuming process due to the number of blood vessels entering and exiting the organ. Each one must be ligated to prevent bleeding. One by one, I dissected out each vessel from the surrounding fat, clamping it close to the spleen's surface and tying it off with 0 PDS. The sturdy suture should prevent any leaks. Over and over, I repeated the process until one last vessel remained.

"Dr. Nelson, she's getting a little pale." I looked up from my work. "And her pulses are weaker," Allie continued. She fidgeted on her stool. Even with her face covered by a cap and mask, I could tell she was nervous. I could see it in her eyes.

"Increase her fluid rate. I'm almost done."

I separated the fat along the border of the spleen and clamped off the artery with a forceps. The vessel throbbed with each heartbeat. This vessel provides blood to the spleen and a portion of the stomach. I threaded suture around the vessel just above the branch supplying the stomach and tied a strong knot. It's a delicate procedure and care must be taken to avoid damaging the stomach's blood supply. The vessel spasmed but did not leak. One snip later, the spleen was free. A large number of silver clamps dangled from its underside as I handed it to Allie. She removed the instruments and slipped it into a plastic bag for histopathology.

"How's she doing?" I asked.

"Her color is about the same, but her temperature is dropping."

"It won't be long now." I needed to close fast but had to inspect the ligatures once more. A bleeder might do her in. The walls of the arteries swelled with each beat of Sugar's heart but the ligatures held. Her stomach remained a healthy pink. Normally, I relax at this stage. But we needed to get Sugar off the table fast. Allie turned the vaporizer dial from 2 to 1.5, lowering the concentration of anesthetic. The race was on.

My hands moved swiftly over the incision. The needle poked down through one side and up through the other. Back and forth, back and forth, until I reunited the edges of the linea alba. Allie stood up, surveyed the incision and turned the dial to 1.0. I felt a bead of sweat form under my cap. Just two layers to go. I tied a knot to anchor the next line of sutures and pushed the needle through the subcutaneous tissue with a needle holder. When the tip emerged, I grabbed it again on the other side. As fast as was sensible, I repeated the motion until I found myself tying a knot at the other end.

"I'm turning her off," Allie said emphatically. She turned the big round dial for the isoflurane until it clicked to zero. Pure oxygen now flowed into Sugar's lungs. I tied the anchor knot for the last layer. In out, in out, the needle passed just below the skin from side to side. With each stitch, the incision grew smaller.

With about an inch to go, Allie stood for another peek. I closed the rest of the incision and pulled the drapes from Sugar's body. Her legs felt stiff and cold, like a dog with frostbite. Even with the heating pad, her temperature dropped to 98 degrees during surgery. I wrapped her limp body in a blanket and carried her to the treatment room. Allie trailed behind with the anesthesia machine and fluids. I stood with Sugar in my arms as Allie retrieved the heating pad from the O.R. I placed Sugar on it and wrapped another towel around her as Allie hung a heat lamp over her.

"Keep her on oxygen until she starts to chew on the tube." I looked into Allie's eyes. "Wait as long as you can to pull it." She nodded and positioned a stool by Sugar. "I'm going to call Ben." I pulled the mask off my face, and it left a red mark over my nose. My skin beneath the mask felt slimy. I pulled off the surgical cap and fluffed my hair. A red line also ran across my forehead from the elastic band.

Five minutes later, Sugar moved her tongue. It flicked from side to side under the tracheal tube. Allie continued to hold the tube in place. A minute later, Sugar coughed and gagged. Allie clamped one hand around Sugar's mouth and the other on the tube. When Sugar coughed again, she pulled the tube from her mouth. Sugar tried to sit up, but couldn't even hold her head up; it flopped back onto the blanket. Allie rolled the dog onto her chest and placed a towel under her chin.

Genny hopped into the treatment room carrying her stump high in the air. She rubbed her face on the I.V. pole, causing the bag of fluids to wiggle at the top. She sat down in front of the cages and stared at the animals inside. A young schnauzer in one of the lower cages sprang to her feet.

"Woof, woof, woof." Unimpressed, Genny limped over for closer inspection. She sat down three inches from the cage, just outside of the pup's reach. "Whoooooooo, whooooooo," the pup cried again.

"Genny," Allie scolded. "Quit tormenting the animals."

Glancing at Allie before returning her attention to the puppy, Genny lay on her side and flicked her tail up and down. The puppy pranced inside the cage. Her nails sounded like pennies in a soda can against the stainless steel. Allie bent down to shoo Genny out of the treatment room. The cat moved just out of her reach and lay down again, still with a view of the puppy. She rolled onto her back with her three legs in the air.

"Genny, knock it off," I ordered upon my return. She jumped up and disappeared under the cages. "How's Sugar?"

"I pulled the tube two minutes ago." Allie pulled up Sugar's lip. "Her color is better and she's starting to shiver."

"And her temperature?"

"She's up to 99 degrees."

I patted Sugar's head. Her entire body shook from the cold. She stared at me through dilated pupils. Nothing seemed to be in focus for her. "Ben will be here to visit in a few hours. Until then, I want you to sleep," I instructed to my marginally conscious patient. "He's very worried about you."

"Bang, bang!" The puppy crashed against the side of her cage. The bowl tipped over, and water sloshed on the floor. Genny retreated back under the cage to get away from the water. Allie instinctively reached under the cages and tried to grab the stubborn cat. Genny ran out the side, back into the pharmacy area. How could such a small three-legged cat possess so much attitude?

The next morning, I couldn't wait for Allie to recheck Sugar's PCV. I drew the blood myself, filled four PVC tubes and loaded them into the centrifuge. With the turn of a switch, the rotor spun the tubes in a circle separating cells from plasma, the liquid component of blood. Sugar ate a little breakfast while the machine roared in the other room. It reminded me of an airplane revving its engines before takeoff.

"Ding, ding," the machine sounded as it clicked off. Sugar looked up from the bowl with food stuck to her whiskers. I closed her cage door. By the time I reached the lab, Allie already held the tube against a white plastic card with horizontal lines across it. "Her PVC is 20 percent! The same as last night." Her smile said it all. For the first time since Sugar's ordeal began, we had something to celebrate. I couldn't wait to call Ben.

By afternoon, the PCV increased to 22 percent. Sugar sat contentedly at the front of her cage and watched other animals. Her appetite returned, along with her interest in the outside. She devoured lunch and begged for more. When Allie ignored her, she barked for more.

Ben and Spice arrived at the clinic for their afternoon visit. Sugar pranced in her cage. She knew what was coming. When she saw Ben and Spice, she tried to jump out of Allie's arms. She wagged her tail and moaned with delight. She felt great, and so did I.

"Looks like the gang's all here," I said taking the seat beside Ben. I patted Sugar and then Spice on the sides of their faces. "Congratulations, Ben, I think she's ready to go home." Ben's eyes glistened. He looked down at his beloved companion. Sugar looked back at him. A pink tongue slipped from her mouth, and she licked his hand. A tear spilled down his cheek, leaving a wet streak on his face.

"Her afternoon PCV is actually higher than this morning by two points," I told him. Ben wiped his face and cleared his throat.

"I, ah, I wasn't sure if I would ever take her home again." He pulled a handkerchief out of his pocket. "She looked so bad ... two transfusions. I thought I was going to lose you, old girl." He patted her head. Another tear ran down his cheek. "Are you sure?"

"If she has any problems, you can always page me." I smiled at Ben and touched his arm. "I want to see her tomorrow to recheck a PCV. If it continues to increase over the next three days, I'll start tapering her medications."

"You're coming home, old girl, you're coming home," he told his dog. Ben held Sugar's head in both hands. She closed her eyes and panted. Spice jumped up and down in Ben's lap, sensing his excitement. Ben released Sugar and looked directly into Spice's little face. "Sugar is coming home, Spice. Your buddy is finally coming home." Spice jumped and licked the bridge of Ben's nose. We both laughed.

"Well, I see Spice agrees with me." I petted her rear end. "It will take us 10 minutes to get all of Sugar's stuff together. Allie will review the medications with you. Call me if you have any questions."

I stood to leave. Halfway to the counter, I stopped and returned to Ben, placing my hand on his shoulder. "Congratulations, Ben. She really had me worried." My voice cracked on the last word. I blinked a few times to clear the tears forming in my eyes.

"Me too." He buried his face in Sugar's fluffy coat, fresh tears flowing down his cheeks. "Me too."

CHAPTER 23

Elvira the Snake

I looked at the snake's head in my hand and wondered how this happened. Desperation set in. The day had started off routinely. I saw appointments, ate lunch, returned phone calls and wrote records.

At 3 p.m., Captain arrived for his last checkup after the car accident. He had healed beautifully. Pink skin completely covered the injured leg, and tufts of hair grew along the margins. He pranced out the front door without a leg bandage for the first time in weeks. It was a moment that makes veterinary medicine worthwhile.

Everything was great ... until Elvira the snake upset her owner, Cheryl. Now here I was sitting cross-legged on the waiting room floor, holding a grumpy snake. I had no idea how to proceed. I waited for inspiration to strike. Professors do not address escaped snakes in veterinary college. Minutes before, people and pets had filled the waiting room. Now empty chairs lined the block walls.

"Dr. Nelson, where are you?" asked a voice from behind the counter.

"I'm over here, Allie." She soon appeared around the corner of the bookshelves. Her purple scrubs looked stunning with her brown hair.

"I heard screaming and ... what are you doing down there?"

"Well, I'm trying to figure out a way to dislodge Elvira from under the door without hurting her."

The boa constrictor had decided she did not like my veterinary clinic. As soon as I finished the antibiotic injection to treat her pneumonia, she made a slither for it. Being an intelligent snake, she headed for the door to the waiting room and poked her head into the space between the door and the threshold. Her plan worked well until she reached yesterday's dinner. The mouse bulging from her midsection stopped the escape about halfway through the door. She wiggled back and forth to free herself but only succeeded in wedging her body tighter.

As the front half of Elvira appeared in the waiting room, women unleashed terrified screams. Society Ladies with fluffy pets, the women wanted no part of an angry boa constrictor. Dogs barked while sinking further into their owner's laps. A cat hissed from his carrier. Two of the ladies ran out the front door, dogs in tow, slamming it behind them. The third took refuge in the kids' area. We heard the Persian cat meow but could see neither him nor his owner.

On the other side of the door, Elvira's owner went into hysterics. She stayed in the exam room with the back half of her snake.

"My plan is to restrain Elvira," I told Allie. "Then the clients will think everything is under control and come back into the building." We both turned to look at the front door. Anxious faces peered through the glass, hands cupped around their eyes. With each breath, the glass fogged beneath their noses. At their feet, a bichon frisé and miniature schnauzer paced, leaving nose prints all over the bottom of the glass. Sunlight danced off the crystals on their fancy leather collars, casting beams of light around their heads.

"I don't think your plan is working." Allie giggled. "You look pretty silly sitting on the floor holding that snake."

This image was not the picture of professionalism advertised by the American Veterinary Medical Association. But what else could I do? I felt my heart race. Never in my wildest dreams did I envision trying to "un-stick" an angry snake. My face turned bright red. I felt stupid.

I looked at the door pinning Elvira in place and considered various options. We could take the door off the hinges. The problem was, each clinic door was made of solid wood and weighed a great deal. If we tried that maneuver, the snake might be crushed in the process. Scratch plan A.

Plan B involved copious amounts of lubrication. With Elvira nice and slippery, she might slide out from under the door. A snake's scales overlap one another in a washboard pattern from head to tail, so if we tried to push her backwards, the scales might be damaged. Because the first rule of medicine is to do no harm, backwards was out of the question.

Besides, the owner would have a fit if anything happened to her snake. She took notable pride in Elvira's perfect scale pattern, showing it off whenever possible.

Backwards was out, but maybe sideways would work. If Allie pulled up on the handle, there might be enough room to wedge her out. I did not have a Plan C.

As I waited for Allie to return with lube, the clinic's front door opened a crack. A black nose surrounded by fluffy white fur poked through the small opening. The nostrils flared several times. Soon another black nose surrounded by grey hair poked through the opening just above the bichon. Both dogs wanted to come inside and investigate this curious smell.

"Is it safe to come in?" the bichon owner asked, still alarmed.

I nodded. "Elvira is a nice snake. She's just upset right now."

"I didn't know there was such a thing as a nice snake," the lady quipped. The door opened and the dogs trotted inside, followed by their owners. The cat owner poked her head out of the children's room but remained in place, content to view the situation from the other side of the front counter. She was not taking any chances.

"Why in the world do you treat snakes?" the schnauzer owner asked. Her face contorted as she spoke. "They give me the creeps."

Although I would not admit to it, I used to have the same reaction. I like lizards and geckos much better. Give me anything with legs. Snakes, especially the big ones, make me uncomfortable until I have control of them. I looked down at the helpless little creature in my hand. Elvira was only three feet long. Over time, I began to feel sorry for snakes. They need medical help, and few veterinarians treat them. That's why I forced myself to overcome my fear and work with them.

"My husband agrees with you," I replied. "He hates snakes. Even a picture of a snake makes him uncomfortable."

Whenever a snake is hospitalized, we cover the incubator with a towel to hide it from view and place a heavy weight on top of the lid to make sure no one escapes. But one heavy bottle is never enough for Steve. When Allie arrived some mornings, she often found the entire top of the incubator covered with gallon jugs, sure proof that Steve did the evening treatments. Poor Steve – I wonder if he would have proposed if he'd known that reptiles were part of the deal. Sometimes it's better to ask for forgiveness than to ask for permission in marriage.

Allie returned with the tube of lubricating jelly. She squeezed a large amount into her hand, knelt down and coated Elvira's body with the clear gel. The ladies watched with a mixture of fear and curiosity. All but the cat owner inched closer for a better view.

"What are you doing?" one of them asked.

"We're putting lube on Elvira, and then we're going to slide her out," I responded. I was not sure if our plan would work, but there was no reason to share that with the ladies. "Allie is going to pull up on the door handle while I slide Elvira out sideways." The ladies frowned. My mother wore the same expression when I told her I wanted to be a veterinarian.

Allie squeezed several more inches of lube onto her finger and painted it on Elvira's scales. The striking browns in her scales stood out like polished stone. Once Allie coated Elvira's entire circumference, she disappeared into the exam room to lube the other side. The back door into the dog exam room squeaked as she entered.

"I can't imagine why anyone would want a snake as a pet," the lady with the bichon reiterated.

"They just lie there in the corner of the cage staring off into space," the schnauzer owner added, adjusting her diamond tennis bracelet. "They even look evil."

"Reptiles and fish are the only pet option for people with allergies," I noted, smiling at the ladies. "And believe it or not, each animal possesses a unique personality." The bichon owner gave me a quizzical glance. "They have likes and dislikes, just like people."

"Oh please, Dr. Nelson," the schnauzer owner disagreed. "Reptiles don't have personalities."

"Sure they do. I know an old iguana named Peaches. She's a big love sponge until she sees a cat. Then, look out. I learned that the hard way." I laughed to myself, picturing Peaches in my mind. I had been carrying her into the back when Genny ran by. Peaches whipped her tail back and forth as she struggled to chase the cat. Her tail wrapped all the way around my body. I had red marks on my skin for two days; it felt like I had been whipped. You can't imagine how much it hurts to shower in that condition.

Everyone laughed. Perhaps my story about Peaches helped them see reptiles in a different light. The ladies moved closer. The dogs pranced behind them, darting between their legs and sniffing the air. I switched Elvira's head to my left hand as my right one started to cramp.

Allie reappeared through the office door. She placed both hands on the chrome door handle and waited for my signal. "All right, Allie, pull up on the door handle and I'll slide her out."

"You mean you hope to slide her out," the schnauzer owner corrected.

"Always confident, often correct," I replied and winked at the group.

Allie pulled with all her might, the muscles in her arms bulging. Her face turned red as she strained. The ladies held their breath, hoping the runaway snake would be freed. I pushed Elvira's body sideways, but it didn't budge. She was wedged tight.

I recalled there was no Plan C.

"Stop; it's not working," I said. "I need more room to maneuver her body." Still holding the snake's head, I sat back on my haunches to re-evaluate the situation. "Just another quarter-inch and it would have worked."

"May we help?" the cat owner asked. She now bravely stood a few feet behind me. The other two ladies nodded in support. Both dogs sat on chairs next to each other, taking in every movement with their keen eyes and ears. They looked like spectators at a football game waiting for the opening kickoff. The cat wisely remained in the kids' area.

"Ah, ah, that would be great," I stammered, astonished by the transformation. A few minutes ago, these ladies ran for their lives. Now they offered to help. "Allie, go inside the exam room and lift from that side while these ladies lift out here. Ask Elvira's owner to help you."

A minute later, everyone was in position. Designer purses sat on the chairs next to the dogs as the three women stood shoulder to shoulder. Manicured fingernails clutched the door, ready to lift with all their might.

"Ready, Allie?" I asked loudly.

Her muffled reply came through the door: "I'm ready, Dr. Nelson."

"On the count of three, one, two, three ... Lift!"

The door creaked as the free end rose about a half inch. I pushed Elvira toward the doorjamb. This time, her body inched sideways.

"It's working!" "Keep lifting."

I continued sliding Elvira until her body rested against the doorjamb. Next, I pushed the thick part of her body backward under the door.

"OK, you can stop now," I instructed.

After everyone let go, I reached up and grabbed the knob. The door swung open, clearing the top of the snake's head with room to spare. Elvira was free! Relief washed over me. I stood up and stretched the snake's body between my hands. Allie needed half a roll of paper towels to remove all of the lube from her scales. Her body looked a little kinked where the door had pinched her. I rotated her from side to side and examined her scales; all of them looked fine. I breathed a sigh and presented Elvira to her worried owner.

The college student inspected her pet for signs of damage, running her fingers over Elvira's body and looking closely at the scales. Satisfied that the pet sustained no damage, she zipped the snake into her black leather jacket. The jacket started to move in unnatural ways. First the zipper bulged, then the back swelled as Elvira searched for another escape route. The jacket looked possessed.

"Elvira!" the owner exclaimed. "Not there!" She unzipped her jacket. The ladies stepped back in utter shock, their eyes fixed on the quivering jacket. Elvira's tail dipped into the owner's pants. The ladies covered their mouths with their hands. I thought they might faint.

"Would you like some help, Cheryl?" I asked.

"No, I've got her," she said. "Elvira does this all the time. She likes to put her tail right down the crease in my butt."

The young woman reached behind her back and removed Elvira's tail, repositioning it around her side. The snake had other ideas. Elvira's tail reappeared in Cheryl's pants as she stood at the counter paying the bill. A look of disgust appeared on the cat owner's face. The schnauzer owner stood motionless with her hand still clasped over her mouth. The bichon owner looked pale. She plopped into a chair, holding her pet close. This was not standard fare for the society crowd.

"Thanks again for taking care of Elvira, Dr. Nelson," Cheryl said. "We'll see you in seven days for the next treatment." She waved and headed outside to a black van. An unnatural silence filled the lobby. As the van pulled away, the ladies erupted.

"Why does the owner use her jacket instead of a cage for transporting the snake? What happens if the snake has to go to the bathroom? Can't you catch disease from a snake? Do the snakes ever bite?"

My head was dizzy from their rapid-fire questions. I explained that I do not recommend transporting reptiles in jackets. I prefer a travel cage with hot water bottles to keep the animal warm. My biggest concern was that one of my patients might get loose in the car and cause an accident. Unfortunately, not all owners comply with a vet's guidance.

"And what about the jacket?" the bichon owner asked. "Why do they put them in there?"

"To keep the animal warm," I replied. "The good news is that I have never heard of one biting while in a jacket." I smiled at the ladies. "I think that shows good restraint on the snake's part." My humor rang hollow.

I decided to ignore the question about defecation. The ladies were already overwhelmed. Because snakes carry salmonella as a normal part of their gastrointestinal flora, an infection from this bacteria is a definite possibility, especially in individuals with weak immune systems. Think of kids who get infected by putting young turtles in their mouths.

I poured sanitizer into my hands from the bottle on the counter. Due to salmonella, I do not support allowing reptiles to roam free in a house. They drag their vents all over, contaminating the environment.

For humans with severe allergies, reptiles and fish are good pet choices. In addition, two other groups of people typically own reptiles. The first is young boys – before they discover girls, that is.

A boy marches with pride into the clinic holding a reptile. After checking in, he sits with the reptile on his lap and offers to show it to anyone who walks in the door. During the examination, he stands close to me and watches everything I do. He asks a lot of questions and tells me all about his pet. His mother, on the other hand, tends to stand in the corner, as far away from the reptile as possible. She shakes her head and often covers her eyes. She seldom speaks.

The other common reptile owner wears black leather and studs and displays a preference for tattoos, body piercings and motorcycles. At first, I thought the snake was just another accessory for the outfit, perhaps a chain substitute. But I was wrong. Most of these people truly love their pets.

"How did the snake get stuck under the door in the first place?" the cat owner asked. I shrugged my shoulders. When I finished working on Elvira, I left her on the table with Cheryl. The snake lay coiled on a warm towel. I don't know what happened after that. I just heard screams.

"The owner told me she decided to let Elvira chill for awhile because the shot upset her," Allie answered. "Elvira slithered down to the floor and under the door before the owner could catch her." She smiled at the ladies. They were not won over. They still thought reptiles should be outlawed as pets.

"Let me clean up the room, and then it's Amici's turn to see the doctor," Allie said. The bichon's ears dropped, and he ran under a chair. He hated coming to the clinic, but I was glad to see him. Plucking hair from his ears sounded great. Elvira was enough excitement for one day.

CHAPTER 24

Chewy the Gerbil

E lvira's unsuccessful escape put me behind on appointments. After the bichon, schnauzer and the cat, the schedule read Chewy, the gerbil. This old gerbil came in every month or so for a teeth trim, a common problem in rodents and rabbits, so I assumed it was time for another trim when I saw her name on the schedule. Sadly, I was wrong.

Billy Carlson adopted Chewy as his fifth birthday present. His parents accompanied him to the local pet store. He surveyed all the possible pets and chose Chewy. From that point on, the two were inseparable. Billy used his allowance to buy Chewy anything and everything a gerbil could want. When Chewy started to lose weight, Billy researched weight loss in gerbils at the library. He looked at her teeth and diagnosed the problem for me.

When Billy entered the clinic, Allie explained that we were running late because of a runaway snake.

"Is the snake still here?" he asked, a concerned look spreading over his face. "Chewy hates snakes. She freaks out if she sees one." He held the carrier under his arm in a protective position.

"No, Elvira's gone, so Chewy has nothing to fear," Allie

responded in a soothing voice. "I have an iguana in back, but no snakes." The boy let out a sigh of relief.

"Please tell Chewy that it shouldn't be too long before her teeth trim," Allie said.

But Billy's mother, Jill, explained that Chewy's teeth were fine. They brought her in because she had started limping on her back leg the previous day. Jill thought it was a sprain and wanted to wait, but her son insisted on a visit to the vet.

The boy held up the plastic crate for Allie. Inside a gerbil stared at her with dark eyes, wrinkling her nose back and forth a few times. The little rodent touched the toes of her back left leg to the ground but did not bear significant weight on it.

Twenty minutes later, Allie escorted Chewy and her family into the dog exam room. When I asked about Chewy, the normally talkative boy remained silent. Jill looked at her son and waited, surprised. Billy sat in the chair with the carrier on his lap, his feet swinging back and forth in the air. His mother answered my questions. When she wasn't sure about the answer, she looked at Billy. He nodded, but still did not speak.

"Other than the limping, is she eating and drinking OK?" Billy nodded. "And she's urinating and defecating normally?" He looked at me with a blank expression on his face.

"Dr. Nelson wants to know if she's peeing and pooping OK," Jill explained. He looked down at Chewy and nodded twice.

When I motioned for Billy to place Chewy on the table, he jumped out of the chair. Chewy stuck her nose through the bars of the door. When I opened it, she sat on her haunches and surveyed the table from the safety of her crate.

"It's OK," Billy whispered. "You know Dr. Nelson; she won't hurt you." Chewy didn't move.

"I think she's worried I'm going to work on her mouth again," I said. At the sound of my voice, Chewy scrambled to the back of the carrier. "See, she's a smart gerbil." Billy beamed with pride, looking up at his mother and smiling from ear to ear. I turned the carrier toward me. "Come here, young lady," I commanded as I stuck my arm inside. Chewy allowed me to scoop her up without a fuss.

Performing a physical examination on a gerbil is the same as any other animal. I started with her head and worked my way back to her tail. Gerbils normally have four big incisors at the front of their mouths. Because these powerful teeth have open roots, they continue to grow throughout life. That means a gerbil can gnaw as much as it wants without fear of wearing out its teeth. Unfortunately, Chewy did not have her upper incisors, only the lower incisors and molars. She stuffed food into the back of her mouth with her front paws. I trimmed the lower incisors every month or so to keep them from interfering with the roof of her mouth.

Chewy cooperated with me until I touched her leg. When my fingers ran over the area between her paw and ankle, she jerked the leg away and turned to face me. She let me feel her knee and hip without complaint but would not let me go any further. The area on her left back leg between her toes and ankle was swollen to twice its normal size. I flipped her over to get a better view. A purple discoloration covered the area on the inner side. Was it a bruise from trauma or something else? I ran through the ruleouts in my mind. None of them were great.

"What do you think it is?" Jill asked, her voice interrupting my thoughts.

"We need to X-ray the leg to see what is going on beneath her skin," I replied. I made a note in her record under the section titled muscular/skeletal system. "She could have a broken bone, an infection or ..." I paused. I did not want to say the last possible cause.

"Or what?" Jill and her son stared at me. I took a deep breath.

"Or cancer." I paused again. "Rodents get a lot of different cancers. Breast cancer is the most common, but I've see other types as well." I waited for the weight of my words to sink in and give them a moment to process the news. "We won't know until we take the X-ray. Hopefully, she sprained her leg, and it will heal with a wrap."

Billy exchanged a worried glance with his mother. He cradled the gerbil with both hands over his heart. I picked up the carrier and held the front toward Billy. He ignored me. I smiled and held the crate a little closer. He turned away from me toward the wall.

"Billy, give Chewy to Dr. Nelson." The boy looked up at his Mom without moving. "William," she said in a firm voice. Billy turned around, kissed Chewy's head and placed her inside. "Don't worry. Dr. Nelson will take good care of her," Jill said as she patted his back and ushered him out of the room. The two headed off to Burger King for a snack while Chewy received her X-ray.

Back in the radiology suite, Allie stood with the technique chart in front of her. The chart contained grids for dogs and cats, but nothing for an animal as small as a gerbil. She studied the prior films of rabbits and birds for guidance. I removed Chewy from her carrier while Allie put on her lead apron and thyroid collar. The brown gerbil crawled up and down my arm, her nose wiggling constantly as she explored her new environment. Chewy was the most well-behaved gerbil I had ever met.

"OK, I'll take the little princess," Allie said as she reached for Chewy. Chewy sniffed her fingers and turned around. Allie looked crestfallen. "What's up? You know you like me better than Dr. Nelson. She's the mean one who trims your teeth, not me."

"But you're the one who holds her for the procedure," I observed. I handed Chewy to her. "I think she remembers your smell." I pulled a second apron off the table, slid my arms into the holes and tied the strings over my abdomen. My shoulders drooped a little under the weight of the heavy garment. Next, I fastened the thyroid collar around my neck with the Velcro ends. Whenever I feel the stiff thyroid collar pinching my neck, I feel sorry for men who have to wear ties to work. I can see why my husband hates them so.

While Allie held Chewy in her arms, I applied two pieces of medical tape to her back legs, encircling her toes with one end and letting the other dangle in the air. Tape handles make it easier to take X-rays of small creatures. With a lead glove over her hand, Allie held Chewy on her side. I teased her legs into position with the tape and covered my hand with a lead shield.

I nodded, and Allie pushed a pedal on the floor with her foot. The machine vibrated and chugged until a loud ding rang. We both let go of Chewy. She rolled onto her side and turned to look at the tape on her feet.

"OK, I'll take them off while Allie develops your film." Chewy crawled into my hand with the strands of tape trailing behind her.

"She really is a good gerbil," Allie remarked. "I hope it's nothing serious."

"Me too," I said.

It took 10 minutes for the automatic processor to spit out Chewy's film. Allie stood in the darkroom with her hand in the tray. When the film cleared the machine, she snatched it and hung it on the viewer in the treatment room.

Because of her small size, Chewy's entire body fit on the film with room to spare. I followed the bones from her skull to her spine to her back legs with my eyes. The bones displayed bright white against the film's black background. As I continued down her leg, the bones looked great until I reached the tarsal area. I could not visualize the many little bones that make up this complex joint because a large mass obliterated the rows of ankle bones that should have been there. The mass seemed to originate from the largest bone in the tarsal joint, exploding from the bone in a starburst.

"What is it, Kris?" Allie asked. She knew from my expression that the prognosis was poor.

"I'm afraid Chewy has cancer," I replied. I continued to scan the rest of the film for other masses. "Based on its appearance, I'm guessing it is an osteosarcoma."

"Poor Chewy." Allie took the news like a professional, but one with a heart. "Why do nice animals with nice owners who will spend money on their pets always get the worst diseases?"

"And mean animals with nasty owners who won't spend a dime on them always live?" I said completing the thought. "I wish I knew."

"It just isn't fair," she continued. The doorbell dinged twice. Allie and I looked at each other. "Are you ready for me to bring them back?"

"No, but bring them back anyway. Waiting won't make it any easier."

Chewy rested in the carrier after her films, her nose poking out a ventilation hole in the side. Her little nostrils opened and closed as she investigated the clinic by smell. The scents from so many animals fascinated her – her nose never stopped moving. She jumped to her feet when she heard Billy's voice. He ran over to the carrier and put his finger inside. Chewy rubbed against it.

"I'm afraid I don't have good news." I paused to collect my thoughts. There was simply no way to sugarcoat my diagnosis. "I'm afraid Chewy has cancer." Billy and his mother stared at me for a minute without speaking. I stood by the viewer and waited for them to respond.

"Cancer," Jill muttered.

"I'm afraid so. Let me show you." Billy and Jill stood in front of the lightbox. The top of Billy's head barely reached my elbow. I pulled the film down to the bottom of the lightbox so he'd have a better view.

"This is Chewy's film. Here is her head," I pointed to the skull. "This is her spine, which continues into this long tail." I ran my finger down her back to the tail. "Now, this is her normal leg." I traced the right back leg. "See all the bones in her ankle?" They both nodded. "Now compare that to the bones in the other leg. You can't see them, can you?"

"All I see is a big white lump," Jill said.

I nodded. "That's the cancer." Jill put her arm around her son and drew him close. Tears ran down the child's face. He sniffled and buried his face in her side. I explained that bone tumors are very aggressive. Treatment starts with amputating the leg and then putting the patient on chemotherapy. Unfortunately, I've never had that cure a patient because this kind of tumor likes to metastasize. It's a nasty cancer.

"What should we do?" Jill asked. "We don't want her to suffer." Billy nodded but kept his face hidden in his mother's side.

"I recommend putting her on an analgesic to control the pain. Then you need to spoil her rotten." I smiled at the pair. "Let her eat all her favorite foods and stay up past her bedtime. Make the most out of the time you have left with her." Jill blinked her eyes several times. She kept one arm around Billy and reached for a tissue with the other.

"How much longer do you think she'll live?" she managed to ask after 20 seconds.

"That's hard to say. With bone cancer, she could have days to months left. It just depends on how quickly it grows and where it spreads."

Jill cleared her throat. She didn't want to put Chewy through surgery and chemotherapy. With her active lifestyle, she felt Chewy would be miserable without her back foot. Instead, they would follow my advice and spoil her rotten. She would be the happiest gerbil on the planet. Billy nodded as tears spilled down his cheeks. They formed a wet spot where he clutched his mom.

"We'll stop at the grocery store on the way home and pick up her favorites," Jill informed her son. I picked up the carrier and held it out to Billy. "Thank Dr. Nelson for helping us with Chewy," Jill coached her son. She unwrapped the child's arms from around her waist and turned him around.

"Thank you, Dr. Nelson," he mumbled, staring at the floor. I smiled down at the child and handed the carrier to him. Inside, I felt like a failure.

"Chewy is a wonderful gerbil," I told him, "and you have done a terrific job taking care of her. Please feel free to call me with any questions or concerns." I put my hand on Jill's shoulder. "I'm sorry it wasn't better news. She really is a special gerbil."

"Thanks, Dr. Nelson," she replied. "We'll be in touch."

CHAPTER 25

Trudy, U.S. Customs Canine Officer

"Welcome to the Minneapolis/St. Paul International Airport," the flight attendant announced after the plane touched down. Static sounded in the background. My legs ached from the lack of legroom. When we reached the gate, I grabbed my bag and stood in the aisle. Ten minutes later, I walked up the gangway into Steve's arms. I couldn't wait to get home.

"Well, how about a ride to the clinic?" Steve asked. I froze in my tracks. A businessman with a large briefcase almost ran into me. "Trudy, the Customs dog, is sick," Steve continued. "The relief vet doesn't know why." He ushered me through the crowded hallway to a quiet corner. "I got a frantic call from Allie this afternoon. I told her to hospitalize Trudy until you arrived."

Trudy, a Lab mix, worked as a drug sniffer for the U.S. Customs Service. Every morning, her handler, Frank Culbertson, picked her up from the boarding kennel next door on his way to work. On this day, Frank and Trudy searched a warehouse in the morning, took a break for lunch and then went back to work. Trudy lay down in the middle of a search and refused to get up no matter what Frank did.

Sensing something was seriously wrong, Frank rushed her to the clinic. The veterinarian who covered for me examined her but couldn't find a reason for her behavior. Trudy just lay there with a sad look on her face. She didn't even try to sniff Genny.

Thirty minutes later, we pulled into the clinic parking lot. A dandelion grew in a crack between the asphalt and the sidewalk. Steve unlocked the front door. I spotted a record with a large note lying on the front counter. Someone had scribbled "Dr. Nelson" on it in bright red ink. I opened Trudy's chart and flipped through the pages. The history section did not give me much to go on. The words "ain't doing right" filled the complaint line on the chart.

"That wasn't very helpful," I said and replaced the record on the counter. Steve turned on the clinic lights even though the sun shone brilliantly through the window. In June, the sun did not set until after 8 p.m.. We Minnesotans view this as our just reward for the long, dark winter nights.

Together, we walked into the treatment room. The stainless steel cages were empty. From the kennel, we heard a dog whimper. Trudy lay in the first kennel run, her black body silhouetted against the gray concrete floor. A rumpled blanket sat in the corner. A small card taped to the gate read "Trudy, U.S. Customs."

I took off my blazer and threw it over one of the empty incubators. Dressed in a business suit, I heard my high heels clip on the floor. I rolled up the sleeves on my silk blouse and donned a surgical gown to protect my clothes.

"Alright, Trudy, time to figure out what's wrong with you," Steve announced. He flipped the latch and swung the gate wide open. Trudy remained on the floor. She thumped her tail a few times, but refused to move. Steve stepped into the run and knelt beside her. "Come on, Trudy, you need to get up now." He put his arms under her chest. She moaned and smacked her lips together. Steve released his grip.

"She won't get up, Kris." He petted her head. "Maybe you should examine her in here?"

"No, the light is bad," I replied. "I need her on the treatment room table." I walked over to her run, hoisted my skirt and stepped into the kennel. "I'll take her chest, and you take her rear end."

"How come I always get the rear end?" he whined.

"Because you're the man," I smiled. I put my arms under Trudy's chest, and on the count of three, we lifted her off the floor in one fluid motion. Trudy looked around sheepishly, her legs dangling as we carried her in our arms. She continued to smack her lips.

Trudy had a long nose, floppy ears and the expressive tail typical of Lab mixes. When she worked, she held her tail straight out behind her. She arched it over her back when she played tug-of-war with her handler. At the clinic, her tail normally moved from side to side in big circular sweeps. Instead of wearing her emotions on her sleeve, Trudy wore them on her tail. Now it drooped behind her. She held her ears flat against her skull as she stood on the table.

Overall, Trudy was depressed. Her hair coat looked dull and lifeless, lacking its normal luster. Her ribs and backbone felt more prominent than I remembered from prior examinations. Her heart rate and respiratory rate seemed higher. Taken together, these symptoms told me Trudy was sick, but not much more. So far, nothing pointed to a problem with any particular body system. She obviously felt horrible, but from what? I rubbed my hand against my forehead.

"What do you think it is?" Steve asked.

"I don't know yet." A frown spread across my face. "Normally, Trudy is a wild child. This is way too calm for her." Hopefully, her blood and urine would tell me something. Before I drew her blood, I decided to perform a rectal examination. I grabbed a disposable glove from the shelf.

Steve wrinkled his nose. "Better you than me."

I slid on the glove and squeezed a blob of lube on my pointer finger. As I slowly inserted my gloved finger, Trudy tried to sit on my hand. Steve placed one hand under her abdomen and hoisted her rear end back into the air.

Bummer, everything felt normal. I pulled my finger out and let go of her tail. Bright red blood mixed with feces covered my gloved finger. "Steve, look at this." I opened a drawer with my other hand and retrieved a glass microscope slide. I pressed the slide against my glove, leaving an imprint of my finger in blood.

Many things can cause bloody feces. I ran through the possibilities in my mind. Gastrointestinal parasites or worms, as many owners call them, damage the mucosa of the intestine. The damaged area bleeds, but usually not this much. She could have a foreign body stuck in her intestinal tract. She is a Lab, after all. I thought of Rusty and his propensity to swallow inanimate objects. Or it could be hemorrhagic gastroenteritis from stress? I pulled the glove inside out as I removed it.

But my gut told me this was a primary bleeding problem; her blood would not clot. Perhaps she ate some rat bait from one of the warehouses. Dietary indiscretion, as we call it in veterinary school, is always at the top of the list with young dogs. I needed to make the diagnosis quickly, or she would bleed to death. I grabbed a syringe and several different blood tubes from the drawer. Steve held Trudy's head up with her neck exposed for a jugular stick. I pointed to her leg instead. It was safer to draw from a smaller peripheral vessel instead of the large jugular vein. Poor Trudy might bleed for a long time.

The dog stood like a statue for her blood draw. Steve held off the vein with one hand and hugged Trudy with the other. I quickly filled several tubes with different colored tops – purple, red, blue and green. One by one, I pulled the rubber stopper out and let the blood trickle down the side of the tube to the bottom. When the red top was filled, I looked at my watch. It read 7:30.

Every minute, I inverted the tube. With normal blood, a soft clot begins to form in two minutes, and all of the blood clots in less than five. If I was right about rat poison, Trudy's blood would take much longer to clot – if it clotted at all.

Steve held a gauze pad over the vein. "Any signs of clotting yet?" he asked. I shook my head back and forth but kept my eyes on my watch. When the second hand reached the two-minute mark, I slowly inverted the tube again. The blood sloshed from one side to the other.

"Be sure and keep holding her leg," I told Steve. "I don't want her to bleed out through the venipuncture site." He readjusted his grip on Trudy's leg.

The seconds continued to tick by. Three, four and then five minutes passed without any signs of clotting. Her blood continued to flow from one end of the tube to the other. I glanced at Steve and Trudy in between inverting the tube. She rested her head on his shoulder. Six, seven, eight, nine and finally 10 minutes ticked by without any clot, even a soft one. "It's been 10 minutes." I placed the tube on the shelf. "I don't think it's ever going to clot."

"Poor Trudy," Steve said as he stroked her head. "What's next? Do we have to make her vomit?"

"No, it's too late for that," I answered. "By the time an animal shows clinical signs, the poison is already absorbed." I searched through the cabinet for bandage material. "I'm going to put a pressure wrap on her leg to keep her from bleeding, and then we'll give her the antidote."

Warfarin is the most common rodenticide in our area. It interferes with Vitamin K1, an important step in the activation of platelets. Without Vitamin K1, the platelets won't aggregate into a clot. A poor animal that ingests this product bleeds to death – a prolonged, awful death. I wish we would find another method for rodent control.

Unfortunately, treating rat bait ingestion is pretty common in practice. The bait appeals to all kinds of animals, not just rats. Some animals come in with bruises all over their bodies. Others bleed from their mouths. In the winter, owners notice bloody urine on the snow. Trudy was the first case I diagnosed from a rectal exam. The bloody stool was her only visible sign of hemorrhage.

The principle behind treatment is simple. Give the patient large doses of Vitamin K1 to out-compete the poison. I grabbed a large needle and syringe. The thick solution burns when injected. I drew Trudy's dose from the brown glass bottle into the syringe.

"Steve, this really hurts," I said. "Let's muzzle her." I grabbed a medium blue one from the rack by the leashes and slipped it over her nose. Trudy did not resist. I injected the irritating solution in multiple sites to lessen the inflammatory reaction. After that, Steve helped me place a catheter for I.V. fluids.

"Good girl, Trudy. You are a brave girl," Steve soothed. "I'll stay with her while you call the officer," he said. I retrieved an office chair for him before heading back to the lobby. Trudy lay down on the table and rested her head on her paws. Steve settled back into the chair with the *Wall Street Journal* in his lap. He placed his arm around her and skimmed the front page.

Frank was waiting for my call; he picked up the phone on the first ring. "Sorry to drag you to the clinic after your trip, Dr. Nelson. I'm sure that's the last thing you wanted to do."

"It's OK, Frank. I'll gladly come in for Trudy."

"So what's wrong with her?'

"Well, I'm afraid she's got a bleeding problem," I replied. "She can't clot. I found blood on the rectal exam, so I did a quick clotting test. In normal animals, the blood clots in five minutes or less. Trudy's blood never clotted."

Silence filled the distance between us.

"What causes it?" he asked.

"Lots of things," I replied. "But I would guess rat poison."

"That can't be. She doesn't have access to any poison." He paused. "What are the other causes?"

"Well, she could have been born with some kind of clotting problem. For example, I always screen Dobermans for von Wille-brand's disease. But Trudy is a mixed breed, which makes that unlikely." I ticked off the causes of bleeding that I learned in school. "She could also have a problem with her bone marrow not making platelets or making platelets that are defective. The list goes on and on." I transferred the phone to my other ear. "But with most of these causes, Trudy would have had problems long before now. She would have bled during her spay." I paused.

"To the best of my knowledge, Trudy has never had any problems like this before," he responded.

"Ever notice any blood on her toys or in her food bowl?"

"No, never."

"That's why I think she has an acquired problem rather than an inherited one. Poison is the most common cause of an acquired clotting problem. This is especially true with young dogs like Trudy. You would not believe some of the things they will eat."

"Is she going to make it?" Frank asked.

"I think so, but of course, there are no guarantees. I've injected her with vitamin K1 and started her on fluids. It will take awhile for the medicine to work. The next 24 hours are critical. If the blood loss doesn't slow down, she might need a transfusion." Frank listened intently and promised to transmit the information to his supervisor.

The next morning, Frank pulled up to the clinic in a new white panel van just as I got out of my car. The windows on the van's back doors were tinted black, and a temporary paper license stuck to the glass. The license plate holder was empty.

"Good morning, Frank," I called from across the parking lot. He turned to face me. He wore a navy blue shirt with large U.S. Customs patches on the sleeve, and his metal name badge reflected the bright morning sunlight. A flashlight, handcuffs and empty holster hung from his black leather belt. He quickly snapped a handgun into the holster.

"Hi, Dr. Nelson," he replied. He grabbed a towel taped into a roll from under the seat and stuck it into the back pocket of his shorts. The seams stretched to accommodate Trudy's favorite toy.

"Did you get a new car?" I asked.

"Yes, we got it in a drug bust last week," he said with a smile. Vehicles and equipment used by drug traffickers became property of law enforcement. The van worked well for transporting Trudy, accommodating her crate as well as other equipment. Frank opened the back door to show off the crate, but the smile vanished from his face as he thought about his dog. He fingered her rolled-up towel in his back pocket. Maybe she would play a little today.

I held the front door open for Frank, but he would have no part of it. He grabbed the door handle and motioned for me to enter first. "Ladies first," he commanded. "Especially when they're treating my partner." I nodded and walked through the open door.

"Good morning, Dr. Nelson; good morning, Frank," Allie greeted us from behind the counter. She handed Trudy's record to me. Trudy's PCV dropped two percentage points overnight. I had hoped it would stay the same or increase slightly in textbook fashion. Unfortunately, Trudy had not read the book.

We took a shortcut through the cat room to the back. The angelfish swam to the front of the aquarium and followed us as we passed. Genny froze against the wall when she saw Frank in the pharmacy area. She didn't like the noise he made as he walked. The squeaky leather and clinking metal alarmed her. The fastest thing on three legs, she scampered into the closet in the office.

"Hello, hello," Bongo greeted us in her feminine voice.

"Hello, Bongo bird," I responded.

"Hello," she said again, this time using her masculine voice. She sounded just like my dad. Frank ignored the greeting. He focused entirely on Trudy.

Trudy drank a little water but refused her breakfast. Saliva dripped from her lips, leaving dark spots on her blanket. She tossed and turned from side to side and occasionally smacked her lips. Her tail hung between her legs, limp and lifeless, she lay in the first run with a bag of I.V. fluids hung above her head. Resting with her eyes closed and her rear end elevated just above her head, she looked like she was praying. Frank's face flashed white when he saw her.

"Hi, Trudy," Frank said in a cautious voice. "How're you doing, kiddo?"

Trudy opened her eyes and wagged her tail once but remained in the same position. I opened the gate and stepped over the threshold. Frank stood outside, not sure if he should enter. I motioned for him to join me inside.

"She's awfully quiet for Trudy," he observed, still standing outside her run. "I've never see her this still."

"Well, her abdomen is really bothering her." I ran my fingers along her sides. She tensed her muscles. When I probed a little deeper, she burped and licked her lips. I waved him into the run again. In slow motion, he stepped over the threshold and knelt beside her.

"Hi, Trudy," Frank said with his fingers buried in the fur around her neck. He ran his hand down her back. Trudy lurched to her feet and circled to the back of the run. She stood with her rear facing us. Frank jumped to his feet and pinned his body against the concrete block wall. He looked at me, frowning. "Is she mad at me?"

"No, I think she's going to vomit," I replied. Right on cue, Trudy's abdomen began to heave. She wretched and deposited a large puddle of foamy material on the floor. The vomitus was a mixture of yellow stomach acid and bright red blood. One long string of saliva hung from her lips.

"Oh, that's nasty," Frank said turning his head away. "I don't know how you guys deal with that kind of stuff."

"We've seen a lot worse," I replied. "Maggots, abscesses and ..." A strange gray-green color spread over Frank's face. He placed one hand on the wall of the run and the other on his abdomen. "Are you OK, Frank?" He nodded but continued to look away.

Vomiting caused by ulcerations along the gastrointestinal tract is a common problem with this kind of poison. It's also very uncomfortable. The night before, I started her on cimetadine to block acid production and sucralfate to act as a bandage for the ulcers. She would feel better once they kicked in.

Giving Trudy one more glance and with his hand still on the wall, Frank announced that he'd better get to work. He stepped out of the run and took a deep breath. "Please let me know if anything changes. I'll be back to see her after work."

"Absolutely," I replied. "We'll see you later."

Despite treatments, Trudy continued to vomit throughout the day. Her PCV dropped a little more but not to a life-threatening level. She felt rotten, and so did Frank. He worried about his partner. His dog's bright eyes and mischievous spirit had evaporated. During his afternoon visit, he placed the rolled-up towel on her paws. She turned away without even sniffing it.

Frank also worried about his job. Questions circled about his handling of Trudy. How did she come into contact with the poison? Did she grab a mouthful of rat poison while working a warehouse? After all, the stuff is used in many of the facilities they search for drugs. Perhaps Frank was not paying attention to her, and she managed to ingest some bait right under his nose. If that was the case, his career as a Customs Department dog handler was over.

The next morning, the landscape crew was hard at work by the time I arrived at the clinic. Grass grew into a lush green blanket under the warm June sun. The smell of freshly cut grass filled the air. Light green buds appeared on the pine trees around the strip mall. I reveled in the sunshine for an extra minute before heading inside. I might not get outside again until after dinner, and I wanted to savor every minute I could.

"I have some messages for you, Dr. Nelson," Allie said. She followed me with a stack of notes in her hands. "Ben called to report that Sugar vomited once last night. She ate her normal breakfast this morning. I told him to watch her and call if she vomits again." She shuffled that note to the back of the stack. "The Siberian husky pup you vaccinated yesterday got into the garbage this morning. The garbage contained chicken bones." I stopped to look at Allie. "The owners will drop her off for X-rays around 10 a.m."

She handed me a business card with the official U.S. Customs logo on the front of it. "And Frank's supervisor wants to speak with you." I nodded and took the card.

I grew increasingly concerned at Trudy's lack of progress.

Overnight, Trudy's PCV fell another point. Her temperature was normal, but she couldn't hold anything down. In my short career, I had already treated many cases of rodenticide ingestion. The patients always responded to treatment and stopped vomiting within 24 hours. I worried there was something else wrong with Trudy.

"Oh, your first appointment is already here," Allie continued. My watch read 8:45. They would have to wait while I checked on Trudy. In the treatment room, I found Genny sitting in front of the cages.

"Genny, no," I commanded. Her eyes widened as she looked at me. "Stop tormenting the patients." She slunk past me out of the treatment room, carrying her stump high off the ground. From the expression on her face, I knew she'd be back again as soon as I left the room.

Through the open door into the kennel area, I saw Trudy lying on a blanket. "Trudy, how are you doing this morning?" She thumped her tail twice. I walked into the kennel area, opened her gate and knelt beside her. Her tail continued to thump up and down in a slow, rhythmic beat. She raised her head and rested it on my lap. I ran my hands over her head and down her back. The top of her backbone protruded from the muscles of her back. There was nothing to pinch over her ribs. All of her subcutaneous fat reserves were exhausted.

"Poor Trudy," I cooed in her ear. She wagged her tail even harder.

"This morning her weight dropped to 42 pounds," Allie announced from the doorway with both hands on her hips. "Frank is really worried about her weight."

"That makes two of us." I stood up and stretched my back. "I think she's less nauseated today. She's not drooling as much." I stepped out of the run and closed the gate. "If you don't see any vomiting by noon, offer her a little water." Allie nodded. "Continue all the other treatments," I said and headed toward the exam room.

The 10 a.m. appointment cancelled at the last minute because the owners couldn't catch their cat. I decided to use the time to call Frank's supervisor. My hand shook as I dialed the number on the card. I always get a little nervous when I speak with government officials.

"U.S. Customs," a man answered.

"Hello, this is Dr. Nelson calling about Trudy."

"Dr. Nelson, thanks for calling. How is our girl doing?"

"Good and bad," I replied. "Her PCV is holding strong, but she's still vomiting." Bongo screamed in the background.

"What was that?" he asked.

"Sorry, that's a mad parrot. It's time for her morning bath." I closed the door to my office.

"What do you think is causing the vomiting?" he asked.

"Well, I think Trudy developed lots of small ulcers along her intestinal tract. Unfortunately, it takes awhile for these to heal. She's getting two medications that should help. I hope ..."

"When do you think she can come back to work?" He jumped in before I could finish. "We need her back ASAP. She's our only drug dog, you know."

"That depends on Trudy, sir," I said. "Once she stops vomiting, she'll need a few days of rest to recover her strength. She should start with short shifts and work up to her normal schedule."

"So it will take about two weeks."

"That's a good guess, but it really depends on Trudy." Allie opened the door and waved her hand at me. "Do you have any other questions?"

"Just one more," he replied. "Any idea how Trudy got poisoned?"

"I'm afraid not, sir," I replied. "We might get a few hints as she progresses through her rechecks, but right now I really don't know."

"Rechecks?" he asked.

"Yes," I replied. "Every three weeks, we'll take her off the vitamin K1 for two days and recheck her blood. If it clots, she's done. If it's prolonged, we'll continue therapy. Some poisons require six weeks of therapy."

"Great, that's the last thing I needed to hear this morning." I heard voices in the background but could not distinguish the words. "Take good care of Trudy, Dr. Nelson. Everybody misses her and wants her back as soon as possible."

"I'll do my best, sir." I hung up the phone and joined Allie in front of the X-ray viewer.

"How did it go?" she asked.

"Fine," I paused. "He wants her back at work."

A film from the garbage-eating puppy hung from the clips. I scanned the chest area first, just in case something stuck in her esophagus or went down the wrong channel into the lungs. Then I shifted to the gastrointestinal system. An enlarged stomach protruded past her rib cage. Inside, gray areas mixed with bits of bright white material – what was left of the chicken. Thank goodness, the pup chewed the bones into little chunks. They should pass through her intestines without any problem. The relieved owners vowed to place a lock on the cabinet to keep the pup out of the garbage. This precocious youngster knew how to open the door with her nose.

At noon, Allie offered Trudy a small amount of water. It had been 12 hours since her last vomiting episode. She sat up on her haunches and wagged her tail. Allie held the bowl under her nose and dipped her fingers in the clear water.

"How would you like a little drink, Trudy?" The dog looked at the crystal-clear water but did not drink. Allie dipped her fingers into the bowl and splashed the water around. Trudy watched but didn't move. She seemed to want the water. What was holding her back? Allie raised her fingers to Trudy's lips and let water drip into her mouth. Finally, the dog began to lick the water off of her fingers. Gradually, Allie moved her fingers closer and closer to the water's surface until Trudy drank right from the bowl. Her bright pink tongue lapped up the water.

"Good girl," Allie praised her. Trudy leaned into Allie's side. Water dripped from the dog's lips onto Allie's leg. She giggled as she brushed the drops off her scrubs. "Good girl," she repeated. "You'll be back at work in no time."

CHAPTER 26

Fourteen Puppies

The first appointment of the afternoon belonged to Abby, a black-colored Labrador retriever. Two days earlier, Abby had given birth to 14 puppies in just three-and-a half hours. From 2 to 5:30 a.m., the experienced mom grunted and groaned to deliver all the pups. Today Abby needed a postpartum exam, and her babies needed their dewclaws removed.

"Congratulations, Abby." I reached under her chin and scratched the new mom's neck. "And to you as well, Jan. I'm sure it was a long night." The slight women nodded. Abby stood by Mrs. Reeves, anxiously eyeing the box on the table. Inside, her puppies slept under a blanket.

"Yeah, we're pretty proud of her," Jan responded. She smiled and pushed her sun-bleached bangs out of her face. A metal barrette held back the rest of her hair. She wore a blue button-down shirt with dogs embroidered on the front and back.

"So, how do you want to do this?" I asked. "The puppies first or Abby?"

"Start with Abby, and then I'll take her out to the truck when you work on the pups."

I nodded and knelt down by the mother. She stood at attention and focused on the box while I examined her. Once in awhile, she snuck a quick glance at me or her owner. I spent a lot of time examining her abdomen, mammary glands and vulva. Everything seemed normal. Milk flowed freely from each gland.

Fourteen is an awfully big litter, even for a large dog like Abby. Right now she probably could produce enough milk for them, but that would change as they grew. In addition, Abby did not have enough nipples to nurse all the pups at one time. Dogs have 10 nipples. The most aggressive pups would nurse at the upper third, fourth and fifth glands. The less dominant would fill in the rest of the spaces, leaving the submissive pups without a place to nurse. Jan supplemented the litter with puppy milk replacer three times a day. I doubled that amount and recommended removing the dominant pups at regular intervals to allow the little ones to nurse.

Although Abby came through the pregnancy in great shape, I worried about her now more than ever. Hypocalcemia or low calcium blood levels, can occur during lactation. If the levels fall too low, seizures occur. I recommended supplementing her diet with cottage cheese and feeding her a mixture of canned and dry puppy food. Having extra calories and calcium would help her avoid any problems.

"Well, she looks great, Jan," I said as I offered Abby a dog biscuit from my pocket. She ripped the treat out of my hand, her teeth grazed my fingers. She wolfed it down in one gulp without chewing. I broke the next two in half and placed them on the floor.

"When do you want us back?" Jan asked. She snapped a lead onto Abby's collar.

"I thought you were going to stay and help me with this?" I'm sure my face reflected my surprise.

"No, I hate it when you remove the dewclaws. Abby and I are going to get a cup of coffee." She looked at Abby. "We'll be back in 30 minutes."

Inside the box, the puppies' bodies morphed into one large pile

of fur, paws twitching as they slept. Several of the smaller ones
sucked on the blanket with their bright pink muzzles. Others
grunted as they searched for a better spot in the group. With their
eyes and ears sealed shut, they used their paws to feel their way
around.

Allie entered the room with a surgical pack, two gowns and an
assortment of other equipment. We washed our hands and slipped
the gowns over our clothes to protect the babies. One by one, we
examined each pup and then removed the dewclaws with a quick
snip. Twenty minutes later, I breathed a sigh of relief when I finished with the last pup. Although I knew that removing their
dewclaws would prevent nail injuries in the field, I still disliked
the procedure.

"Dr. Nelson, we've got a bleeder on this pup." Allie held up a
large male. "He needs a little more glue on this paw." I wiped away
the blood and squeezed one drop of blue tissue glue onto the area.
We watched the incision for 30 seconds, and this time, the glue
held. The beautiful black pup slept in Allie's hand like nothing had
happened.

"I'm glad I'm not Jan," Allie said as she covered the pups.
"She's in for some sleepless nights."

"Or Abby," I added with a wink.

When Abby and Jan returned, the dog ran straight through the
door to her puppies. Jan removed the blanket and held the box
down at her level. Abby sniffed each puppy from head to toe. She
did not like the glue holding each incision closed. She rolled the
largest puppy on his back and tried to lick all of it off.

"No, Abby," Jan scolded. She pushed Abby's face out of the box
and replaced the blanket. "You can clean them when we get home."
Jan picked up the box and headed out the door with Abby close
behind. Animal moms are remarkable. She was not going to let
those puppies out of her sight again. Allie escorted them to the
parking lot.

As Jan loaded Abby and her puppies into her truck, a car raced

into the parking lot. Allie recognized the driver instantly. It was
Paula Anderson, owner of Sadie and Maggie. Something must be
terribly wrong for Paula to drive so fast. She always seemed to be
the careful, meticulous type.

The car squealed to a halt in the handicapped spot in front of
the clinic. Paula threw open the door and ran to the passenger side
where she picked up Sadie. Holding her head in an unnatural position, it appeared the cocker spaniel did not know which way was
up.

"Paula, what's wrong with Sadie?" Allie asked.

"I don't know," the owner said quickly. "She was fine when I
left for work this morning." Tears rolled down Paula's cheeks. "But
when I got home, she was like this. I think she had a stroke." Her
voice cracked.

"Bring her right in." Allie ushered her through the front door
straight into the cat room. "Dr. Nelson, we need you now," she
yelled.

Paula bent down and placed her beloved pet on the table. Sadie
immediately tried to roll off, flinging her body to the side. Her legs
pawed the air. Her eyes oscillated in their sockets – she looked possessed. Allie grabbed her rear legs and pinned them in place. Paula
held Sadie's head between her hands and cradled the body between
her forearms. She put her face in Sadie's fur and sobbed.

"Oh dear," I muttered as I entered the room. The words escaped
my mouth before I could suppress them.

"She was like this when I got home from work." Paula was
frantic. "She rolled herself into the wall and was stuck there." Tears
spilled down her face onto the table. "Did she have a stroke?" she
whispered.

"No, I don't think so." I put my hand on her shoulder. "I think
she has a problem with her middle ear. Let Allie take her front end,
OK?" Paula slowly released her grip on Sadie. Drawing the dog
toward her, Allie placed one arm under the dog's abdomen and the
other around her neck, using a hand to hold Sadie's head against

her shoulder. Paula stood on the other side of the table, not knowing what to do.

"See how her eyes are moving back and forth?" I asked Paula. I turned Sadie's head to the side for Paula to see. "Her eyes drift to the right and then snap back to the left. See that?" She nodded. "This is termed nystagmus. It tells me that Sadie has a problem with the right side of her vestibular system." I looked down her ears with an otoscope. Both canals were free of debris. The eardrums looked great.

"Older dogs get idiopathic vestibular syndrome," I noted. I continued with Sadie's examination while explaining the condition to Paula. "The vestibular system is what gives us our sense of direction. Right now, poor Sadie doesn't know which way is up. That's why she's contorting her body into these weird positions."

"Is there any hope for her?" Paula sniffled and blew her nose.

"Yes, many dogs recover from this condition."

"Really?" For the first time, Paula looked at me with hope, not dread, in her eyes.

"I know this looks bad right now, but I've had good luck treating these cases," I said. I petted Sadie's head. "We're going to give her supportive care for tonight. Right now she's really nauseated, so she won't eat or drink. Tomorrow we'll pursue further diagnostic work."

"So she'll stay in the hospital tonight?" Paula asked.

"Yes, most of the animals with this condition stay in the hospital for a few days," I said.

"Maggie is going to go crazy without her," the owner replied. "These two are inseparable."

"Don't worry," I soothed. "I'll give you some tranquilizers for Maggie." I motioned for Allie to take Sadie in back. "Give Maggie one as soon as you get home and then another before bed. That should get her through the night without any problems."

"Can I take one, too?" Paula asked.

"Sorry, you're on your own." I squeezed her arm. "I promise to call if anything changes."

"Thanks, Dr. Nelson, please take good care of her," Paula said. "You have no idea how traumatic this is. I'm going through a divorce. I just can't lose her now."

"Hang in there, Paula," I said. So often, other events in people's lives are magnified during times of medical crisis. It only added to the pressure I felt to help Sadie recover.

At 5 p.m., I sat down in the office to catch up on paperwork. A six-inch stack of records occupied one side of the desk; Genny took up the other. Her beautiful tortoiseshell markings matched the teak wood perfectly. Although I enjoyed her company, she left me no room to work.

I pulled the first record off the pile and laid it on my lap. The label on the front cover read "Sadie Anderson." I flipped to the examination sheet and made notes in the medical history and physical examination sections. In the short time since her admission to the hospital, Sadie seemed less disoriented. Her nystagmus slowed from 10 oscillations in 10 seconds to five. She still held her head in a twisted position, but wasn't rolling anymore.

Under the treatment plan category, I made the following note: "Sadie is responding well to conservative therapy. Continue with supportive care overnight. Consider further diagnostics tomorrow as warranted by her condition. Keep her cage padded to prevent injury if she starts to roll again. ****Do not leave her alone with the I.V. line attached. Monitor closely to make sure she does not entangle herself in the line. Owner was notified that Sadie is progressing faster than expected."

I closed the chart and dropped it to the floor. Genny jumped when it hit the ground. One by one, I continued to update the records on my desk. Business was picking up. I was so grateful, and Steve's stress about the practice seemed to be abating. I welcomed the increase in revenue, but with it came a decided increase in paperwork. With two records to go, Allie stopped by. In her hands were a bowl and a tongue depressor.

"Dr. Nelson, I'm fixing Trudy's dinner," she said, tilting the bowl toward me. Inside I saw two chunks of canned dog food, about a quarter of a cup total. "Is this enough?"

"That's plenty for her first meal." I stood up, and so did Genny. She stood facing the bowl with her nose high in the air. "I sure hope she eats this!" I said.

"Me too," Allie echoed. "Me too." Allie used the tongue depressor to break the two chunks into smaller pieces as we walked back to the kennels. Genny jumped from the desk to the chair to the floor and followed us. Every few steps she stopped and sniffed the air again. If ever a cat was precious to observe, this stunning three-legged beauty was it.

When we reached the kennel, Genny stopped at the doorway and rubbed on the doorjamb. The friendly Samoyed next to Trudy started to bark and whine. Genny sat down and looked at him with utter disdain, casually licking her paw and rubbing her ear. She took a sinister delight in reminding other animals that they were behind bars. The dog moaned and spun in circles in his run.

"Time for dinner, Trudy," Allie announced as she opened the door to the run. Trudy rolled up onto her side and blinked. Allie held the bowl out in front of her. When the aroma of the food hit Trudy's nostrils, she sprang to her feet and shoved her face into the bowl, almost knocking it out of Allie's hands. Two gulps later, Trudy looked up with ears at attention. She clearly wanted more. She licked the bowl and continued to beg.

"May I give her a little more, Dr. Nelson?" Allie asked.

I shook my head to emphasize the point. "No, that was plenty. She'll get more if she holds this down."

Genny stood on her hind leg with her front feet over the block threshold. She looked around for a minute and then jumped right into Trudy's run. Trudy sat down, a puzzled look on her face. Genny stood on her one back leg, placed one front leg on Trudy's neck for balance and the other on the dog's face. She licked the corner of Trudy's mouth.

"Genny!" Allie exclaimed. "That's Trudy's dinner. I'll feed you next." She picked Genny up and closed the gate behind her. Genny struggled in her arms and complained loudly. "I don't know how to tell you, Dr. Nelson, but you and Steve raised a brat." Genny continued to meow.

"It wasn't us," I replied. "Blame it on my parents. They undid all of our good training when she stayed with them."

"Yeah, right," Allie responded. She placed the matron of the clinic back on the floor. Genny's eyes flashed with anger. She sauntered over to Allie, swatted her leg and then scampered away. I erupted in laughter. Allie was not amused. "See what I mean?"

Trudy stood on her back legs with her front feet braced against the gate. She barked loudly twice, making both of us jump. When we looked at her, Trudy swung her tail in enormous arcs. Her entire rear end swayed back and forth. Joy has seldom been expressed with such eloquence.

"See, even Trudy agrees with me." Allie reached over the gate and petted her head. Trudy continued to wag her tail. She felt great. Trudy, Officer of the U.S. Customs Service, was coming back!

CHAPTER 27

Cow Doc

At precisely 9 a.m., Frank walked through the front door with Trudy at his side. She pranced into the clinic, eager to see her friends, her black fur glistening in the sunlight. In the three weeks since her hospital stay, Frank slowly worked Trudy back into her normal duties. Now he eagerly awaited this recheck, hoping they could put the long ordeal behind them.

"Good morning, Allie," he said. Without waiting for a reply, he marched Trudy straight to the scale. She pranced onto it. "Stay," he commanded with a seriousness reflecting his role as a law enforcement officer. Trudy froze and locked her eyes on his face. The numbers on the digital display bounced around for a few seconds. It stopped on 47 pounds, almost her normal weight. So far, her recovery was right on target.

At Frank's signal, Trudy jumped off the scale into Allie's arms. The dog's ears flopped back against her head, her mouth open in a silly grin. Allie ran her fingers through Trudy's coat and scratched the area under her collar. Trudy closed her eyes and savored the moment.

"OK, let's go draw your blood. Follow me," Allie said. She

escorted Trudy and Frank into the pharmacy area. Trudy heeled by his left leg, her eyes darting around the room and her tail waving back and forth. She wanted to explore, but the highly trained canine that she was, she stayed in perfect heel position.

"Hello, Frank, it's good to see you again," I said, shaking his hand. "And Trudy, how are you?" Trudy looked up at Frank and waited for a signal. Her tail continued to wag at warp speed. Once he gave her a sign, she jumped toward me with a wild grin on her face. I wrapped my arms around her. "Well, I'm glad to see you, too." She looked into my eyes and licked me silly.

As the blood test processed, Trudy zipped around the clinic. She stopped in front of the treat jars and waited for Allie to give her one. When the dog finished exploring, she returned to the pharmacy and lay down next to Frank. Genny caught a glimpse of her from her perch on the office desk chair. She sauntered over and sniffed Trudy's body from head to toe. Trudy looked at Frank for guidance. She couldn't understand Genny's forward behavior.

"Trudy, you remember Genny, don't you?" I smiled, showing my dimples. "She tried to steal your food, remember?" Trudy got up and stood behind Frank's legs. This big brave dog that searched warehouses and luggage carousels was visibly uncomfortable around my little cat.

When the timer read five minutes, I picked up a small tube marked "Trudy" from the test tube rack. Slowly, I inverted the tube. Trudy's blood sloshed down to the other side. It was still liquid. My heart quickened as I repeated the process. Each time I inverted the tube, blood ran from one end to the other without any signs of clotting.

"I'm afraid she's not clotting, Frank." His face blanched. I showed him the tube. His jaw quivered ever so slightly as he watched the blood inside. He took off his gold-rimmed glasses, wiped them on his shirt and replaced them.

"But she seems fine." He cleared his throat. "You can treat her, can't you?"

"We need to start vitamin K1 immediately, or she's going to bleed again." Frank looked down at Trudy, his eyes brimming with tears. Trudy sensed something was wrong. She searched his face, rubbed her body against his leg and nuzzled his hand with her nose. "I'm going to inject her again just to be safe. I want you to start the capsules tonight."

"But she's going to be OK, right?" he pleaded. "I mean, did we catch it in time?"

"Yes, we caught it in time." I looked at the tube again. At 10 minutes, the blood still ran like water. "I've never seen one before that didn't clot at all after three weeks. I've had a few with prolonged clotting times but never one that didn't clot at all." I inserted the tube back into the rack. "She got into some nasty, nasty stuff."

Frank held Trudy as I injected her with the vitamin. The thick solution flowed slowly through the syringe. Trudy squirmed but did not try to bite. With the antidote administered, she climbed into my lap and cuddled. Trudy needed time for the vitamin K1 to kick in. I instructed Frank to give her two days of rest before starting half days again.

"We were supposed to inspect several flights this afternoon," Frank replied. A somber mood spread over him. "My boss is not going to like this."

"Well, tell him to call me if he has any questions. But I don't want her to work today, especially the luggage carousels. It's just too risky."

"OK," he replied. "Trudy's health comes first."

After Frank left the clinic, I headed to the office for my scrubs. Allie had blocked off most of the morning for surgery. Interesting cases filled the schedule.

Cleopatra Davenport was up first. Stacy had found another mammary gland tumor on the little poodle's body. Although this tumor was smaller than the previous ones, it struck me as more aggressive. Many blood vessels grew into it, and the skin in the area had a strange purple cast. The skin looked like it was ready to rupture.

When I emerged from the bathroom, Allie stood next to the treatment table. The clippers buzzed in her hand as clumps of white fur fell to the floor. Cleo lay on her back with a tracheal tube down her throat as monitors beeped around her. A few wisps of brown hair protruded from Allie's surgical cap. A mask tied only by the bottom strings hung from her neck, swinging back and forth over Cleo as Allie worked. The radio played rock and roll in the background.

"I can transfer Cleo myself, if you want to start scrubbing," she said, continuing to work.

"Is that a hint?" I asked.

"Maybe," she smiled. "I would love to finish surgeries on time for a change."

The instant Allie stopped speaking, the phone rang. She frowned and snapped off the clipper. I waved her off.

"Minnesota Veterinary Center, how may I help you?" I answered without identifying myself.

"Kris," the feminine voice answered. "Is that you?"

"Hi, Melanie," I replied. "What did Rusty eat this time?" Allie looked up and laughed.

"Kris, I'm not calling about Rusty," she said, slightly perturbed. "Rachel is sick. Her pediatrician doesn't know what's wrong." Her voice trembled. "I'm sorry to bother you, but I didn't know who else to call."

For the past two months, Melanie's daughter had suffered severe bouts of diarrhea, soiling her bed every night. I cringed at the thought. She had lost 10 pounds and looked like a walking skeleton. Her pediatrician ran all kinds of tests on her, but found nothing. The standard anti-diarrheal drugs were of no use. She woke up in a mess every morning.

"Now they want to anesthetize her for another series of tests." Melanie's voice trembled even more. "She's so thin, I'm afraid she's going to ..."

"What medications has Rachel been on?" I interrupted her.

Melanie rattled off a list of different drugs. When the trade name was unfamiliar, I asked her to read the generic. I hoped the past drug failures would help me rule in and out possible causes.

"Melanie, did the pediatrician check for Giardia?"

"Uh, I don't know," she responded. "What's Giardia?"

That year, I diagnosed more animals with Giardia infestations than ever in my career. The waterborne intestinal parasite causes horrible diarrhea in animals and humans. It's often seen in individuals who drink unpurified stream water when hiking. I suspected the heavy spring floods had contaminated our drinking water.

Allie pushed the anesthetic machine into the O.R. with Cleo in her arms. I pressed my body into the wall to get out of her way.

"I don't think it's that because they've checked her stool several times and never found anything," Melanie replied.

"I know, Melanie, but since human parasites are so rare in the U.S., our physicians aren't the best at finding them unless they have third-world experience," I said.

The organism can be hard to diagnose. Traditionally, the discovery is made from a fecal sample. Unfortunately, the kite-shaped organism is difficult to spot because of its small size and transparent appearance. In addition, the organism is shed intermittently. Depending on the stage of infection, there could be thousands or none in the sample. A veterinary company is working on a snap test that will make diagnosis more straightforward.

"Until a better test is available, I sometimes run a therapeutic trial," I said.

"A therapeutic trial," she repeated. "What does that mean?"

"It means you give the drug and see if the diarrhea responds." The line went silent. "Melanie, if I were you I would run a fecal sample on Rusty. Since Rachel and Rusty are inseparable, I think Rusty might give us the answer to Rachel's condition."

"You know, Rusty had some diarrhea awhile ago. I just thought he ate something again but ..." She paused. "It was about the same time Rachel started soiling the bed. I never put the two together."

"I'm not 100 percent certain that's what Rachel has, but I sure am suspicious," I replied. Allie motioned to me through the O.R. window. "Well, I need to scrub for surgery. Get a fresh stool sample from Rusty and bring it right in for ..." I heard the phone click, and the line went dead. Melanie was on her way. "... a fecal analysis." I hung up the phone. It was time to work on Cleo.

Now that Stacy knew how to check for breast cancer in dogs, she checked Cleo all the time. Every evening, she felt Cleo's body while they lounged in bed. Lady lay next to them and waited for her turn. Last night, Stacy noticed the bruised area on Cleo's mammary gland and tossed and turned all night, worrying about the new lump. She wanted it off immediately.

When Allie had arrived at the clinic, Stacy was waiting outside with Cleopatra dressed in a pink sweater. Cleo seemed to like the sweater even in our hot, humid weather of July. This time I took the entire gland when I removed the lump. Allie placed the excised tissue in a large specimen cup filled with formalin and wrote "Cleopatra Davenport" on the label.

Because of their small size, poodles lose body heat quickly. Poor Cleo shivered uncontrollably as she woke. I wrapped her in towels warmed in the dryer and placed her in the incubator. While Allie set up the O.R. for our next patient, I sat with Cleo to monitor her recovery.

"Ding, ding," the doorbell chimed from the pharmacy. I instinctively knew who it was.

"Allie, Melanie is here with a stool sample on Rusty."

Ten minutes later, Allie marched into the treatment room. She almost stepped on Genny who was playing with a dust bunny. "Dr. Nelson, you were right!" she exclaimed. "Rusty has Giardia." I smiled with relief. "His stool stunk to high heaven. I found it on the direct. He was loaded with them."

"Draw up some metronidazole for him," I instructed. "Tell Melanie I'll be out to talk to her in a few minutes."

"Too late, Dr. Nelson," Allie replied. "She took off as soon as I told her the results. She's on her way to the pediatrician's office. Her husband will swing by for the meds on his way home from work."

"I guess I would do the same thing if my kid was soiling the bed every night," I agreed. "How is Rachel?"

"She looks awful," Allie observed. "And she didn't get into trouble like usual. She just sat in a lobby chair." I shrugged. Like Rusty, Rachel never sat still. She must be really sick.

We finished our final surgery in record time. I pulled off the surgical gown, crumpled it into a ball and tossed it into the dirty clothes basket. With all the patients doing well, we could finally eat lunch. I grabbed mine and settled down in the office. Halfway through a sandwich, Allie burst into the room. Rachel's pediatrician was on line one and demanded I speak with him immediately. I picked up the receiver, took a deep breath and hit the button for line one.

"Hello, this is Dr. Nelson." Allie stayed by my side.

"What the hell do you think you are doing, treating one of my patients? I'm going to report you to the board. You can't practice medicine without a license." The hair on the back of my neck stood up.

"Excuse me, but Melanie Baylor called me for help because you couldn't diagnose her daughter. I told her the condition sounded a lot like Giardia. Since the spring floods, veterinarians have seen a great deal of it." I paused to catch my breath. "I only got involved because she asked me."

"It doesn't matter what she said or did," he replied, flustered by my answer. "You have no right to tell her about Giardia or recommend a therapeutic trial. I'm Rachel's doctor, not you," he said, still screaming into the phone.

"And I'm Rusty's doctor. We just found Giardia on his fecal sample. Did you check for Giardia?"

"Of course I did, you idiot. I ran a fecal. The results were negative." He continued to mutter. I worried the doc would induce his own coronary event.

"Which test did you run?" Silence filled the line. I waited for five seconds before continuing. "Giardia can be difficult to diagnose. It's often missed on routine fecal analysis. You need to do a fecal smear to find the kite-shaped organisms." He started to speak, but I kept going. "Or an antigen test when it becomes available. That's why we sometimes use therapeutic trials in veterinary medicine."

"I'm not taking advice from a cow doc," he shouted. "If you apologize, I might forget you ever did this."

"And when the test comes back positive, I expect an apology from you," I replied. The doctor gasped. "And don't blame the dog for this, either. I'm tired of ignorant pediatricians falsely accusing..."

Bam! The pediatrician slammed the phone before I could finish. I pulled the receiver away from my ear. It echoed from the loud noise.

"What did he say?" Allie asked mischievously. "What did he say?"

"He said he wasn't taking advice from a cow doc." I replaced the receiver with one hand and rubbed my ear with the other. "And he threatened to file a complaint against my license for interfering with his case." Now a mixture of anger and concern filled Allie's eyes.

"Well, Melanie wouldn't have come to you if he had diagnosed it." Her face turned red.

"That's what I told him." I continued to rub my ear. "He didn't take it too well."

"But what if he reports you?" Allie bit her lip after she spoke.

"No worries, Allie." I winked. "I never prescribed medication or diagnosed Rachel. I just said I've seen a lot of it in animals, so I would recommend testing for it." It's a shame the human and veterinary fields do not have closer ties. Zoonotic disease with the ability to pass between humans and animals should make it imperative.

I grabbed a stack of messages and lab work sitting by the counter. "That guy, and more importantly Rachel, are lucky Melanie thought to ask," I continued as I walked back to my office. "Remind me to call Melanie tomorrow for an update." Allie nodded and ripped a piece of paper off the tablet she always kept in her pocket.

The next morning, Allie waited behind the counter for me when I entered the office. She looked at her watch and pointed at its face to highlight my late arrival.

"Oh, cut it out," I laughed. "It's only 11 a.m."

The night before, my pager went off at midnight for a kitten who bit an electric cord. The poor thing had a burn mark across the roof of her mouth. Her lungs filled with fluid, and she couldn't breathe. I did everything I could, but nothing helped. She died at about 2 a.m. Watching the kitten struggle for breath was torture. I paced around our townhouse for two hours before exhaustion finally took over at 5 a.m.

"Is there anything that needs my immediate attention?" I asked Allie.

"No, everything is under control," she responded. She pushed her glasses back into place. "Cleo nibbled on her breakfast this morning. She's a bit more swollen today."

"That's normal, especially with glandular tissue." I smiled at Allie. "Any messages?" She handed me four scraps of paper. When I started to thumb through them, she cleared her throat and stared at me. When I did not respond, she cleared her throat again, her eyes brimming with mischief. She had one last message to share.

"Melanie Baylor called." I stopped thumbing through the notes. "Rachel has Giardia. The lab found it when they did the proper test."

"So the cow doc outdiagnosed the pediatrician," I shouted. Vindicated by the lab, I could hardly contain my enthusiasm. I pictured the pediatrician's face as he read the lab results.

"Do you think he'll call to apologize?" she asked.

"No, his ego won't let him," I replied.

"What a jerk," Allie muttered. "He'll probably try to blame the whole thing on the dog."

"I warned him not to do that," I reminded her.

"But what if he does? I suppose some owners might abandon their pets because of faulty advice from the likes of him."

"If he does, I'll report him to the board and recommend parasitology C.E. He's a disgrace to the pediatric community." I tucked the notes in my pocket. "How was Melanie?"

"Relieved," Allie declared. "How long will it take for the diarrhea to stop?"

"I don't know about humans. But if they respond like animals, Rachel should be back to normal within a few days." Then a deliciously wicked thought entered my mind. "A few days, that is, if the doc gets the dose right."

CHAPTER 28

Emergency of the Male Variety

August is the last month of predictably warm weather in Minnesota. Before school starts, families head to lake cabins to frolic in the warm summer sun. Many travel to Duluth to enjoy the north shore of Lake Superior. Unfortunately, these outings often lead to injuries for the animals.

Beep, beep, beep, the pager sounded from the nightstand. I opened my eyes and stared at the clock. Eleven thirty glowed from the digital display. Beep, beep, beep. I threw back the sheet, sat on the edge of the bed and dangled my feet over the side. Beep, beep, beep. I grabbed the pager and squinted at the number illuminated on the panel.

"Who is it?" Steve asked. A big black cat rested between us, his eyes glowing in the moonlight streaming through our bedroom window. The hum of the air conditioner drowned out the crickets and other night creatures.

"I don't recognize the number." I stretched and yawned. "I need to turn on the light, so cover your eyes." Steve swung his arm over his face. I twisted the knob on the lamp, and light flooded the bedroom. The cat blinked his eyes and looked away. His diamond-shaped pupils narrowed to a slit.

"Hello, Reeves' residence," a feminine voice answered.

"Jan, is that you?" I asked, still not fully awake.

"Yeah, it's me." She paused and giggled. "I'm not sure if this is an emergency or not, so I thought I'd better call." She giggled again. "You remember Abby and the 14 puppies?"

"Yes," I replied and rubbed my eyes.

"Well, tonight when I checked on them before bed, I noticed ..." She laughed nervously. "Well, I noticed one of the pups had ah, ah ,ah." She paused. "Well, his ah, ah, ah."

"Yes," I responded, trying to encourage her.

"His wiener is twice the size as normal," she blurted out. "Is he being naughty already?"

"Naughty," I repeated trying to decipher what she meant. My head felt like it was full of mush. "Naughty," I repeated again. "Are you asking if this is an erection?"

She laughed nervously but evaded a direct answer. "He is moaning and rolling around on his back. I think he might be in pain but Tony thinks he's just having fun."

"Well, there is a condition in dogs where the penis gets stuck in the out position. I've seen it occur in newly weaned pups."

"Oh my God, we just weaned them yesterday," she responded.

Paraphimosis occurs when a male cannot retract his penis into the preputial sheath. The preputial opening acts like a rubber band around a finger, blocking the normal blood supply. The penis becomes more and more painful as it swells. If the penis is not returned to its normal position quickly, permanent damage may occur.

When the pups are taken from their mom, they search for something to suck on that resembles a mammary gland. They sometimes confuse the tip of the penis for a nipple. Usually it's the most submissive puppy in the litter who becomes the victim.

"What color is his penis?"

"It's purple."

"That's bad, Jan. I think the prepuce is cutting off the circulation to his penis. He needs emergency care. He's in a lot of pain."

"Geez," she replied. "We have the worst luck."

"Do you have some KY jelly?"

"Yes, I think so."

"Good, rub that on his penis to keep it moist and meet me at the clinic. I'll be there in 15 minutes."

Steve and I drove through the side streets of Burnsville. We rolled down the windows to let the night air wash over us. A full moon illuminated the night sky, almost erasing the stars and flooding the landscape with shimmering light. We drove to the clinic in silence, each lost in the beauty of the harvest moon and each tired, very tired.

A half-ton pickup with an empty gun rack resting across the back window pulled into the parking lot behind us. A small decal of a hunting dog on point adorned the lower corner, below the rack. Lettering on each door spelled out "On Point Kennels" in big green letters with a phone number for further information. A stout man with sun-bleached hair climbed down from the truck, walked around to the passenger side and opened the door. Jan handed her husband a handsome black puppy with brown eyes and a jet-black nose.

"I sure hope we didn't drag you out of bed for nothing, Doc," Tony grunted.

"Well, we'll know in a flash." I smiled and unlocked the front door. Steve held it open while I flipped on the lights.

"Please follow Kris," Steve instructed.

I led them behind the counter through the doorway into the pharmacy area. When I turned on the lights, the birds ruffled their feathers under the cage covers. Tony snapped his head toward the unexpected sound.

"What kind of birds have you got here?" he asked.

"Pets, no game birds," I replied, having a little fun. "A parrot, canary, lovebird and a cockatiel." I smiled at Tony.

In the treatment room, I motioned for him to place the puppy on the table. The large belt buckle on Tony's waist depicted a hunting scene. A man dressed in camouflage pointed a gun at the sky while a Labrador retriever flushed pheasants from a bush. The ornate buckle left white wear marks in his jeans. Jan stood behind him with a sheepish look on her face. I detected a faint smell of alcohol in the air.

"OK, let's take a look." Tony peeled the towel off the pup and rolled him onto his side. "Oh my," the words escaped my lips. The pup's penis was four times the size I expected. It looked like a large purple sausage with the prepuce cinched around the base. "The poor pup," I whispered. "This is the worst one I've seen."

"See, I told you Tony," Jan proclaimed with the confidence of a woman in the right. "I told him this was abnormal."

Steve peered over my shoulder and winced at the sight. The puppy arched his back and let out a loud cry. He swung his head toward his rear end, but I blocked him from reaching his target. Licking would only make the situation worse.

Because of his young age, I decided to anesthetize the puppy using only gas. If something went wrong, I could remove the nose cone and wake him up. I didn't have that luxury with injectable drugs. Once they were in the patient's system, it was out of my control.

Steve held the furry pup close to his side while I set a catheter in his front leg for fluids. Next, I placed the small nose cone over his muzzle and turned on the gas. The little guy wrinkled his nose from the strange smell. He moaned a few times, then drifted off to sleep.

Steve repositioned the pup's limp body on a towel with his abdomen toward me. I slipped my gloved hand under his penis and gently lifted it up for a better look. The edges of the prepuce cut deeply into the sides of the penis. It was so tight that I could not even get my finger nail to pass through.

"OK, it's time to shrink the beast," I announced.

"How are you going to do that?" Jan asked.

"I'm going to coat it in dextrose. The sugar will draw out the inflammation." Steve handed me a clear plastic bottle of 50 percent dextrose. The rubber stopper popped like a champagne cork when I pulled it from the neck of the bottle. Tony whispered something to Jan that caused her to giggle. Next, I placed a paper towel under the pup's penis and poured. The thick liquid crawled down the neck of the bottle, hung in the air for a second and then dripped onto the target.

"How long does it take?" Jan asked boldly. She stared at Tony as she spoke. He looked like a husband who was in the doghouse. He stood quietly with his shoulders slumped forward and his hands shoved deep in his pockets. Tinges of pink appeared on his face.

"About five minutes in normal cases," I answered. "But hard to say with this one."

For 10 minutes, we watched and waited. Trying to break the tension, Tony shared stories from field trials he completed last week. As he ticked off the accomplishments of his dogs, I noticed the swelling slowly recede. The deep purple color melted into an angry pink.

"Look," I pointed at the pup. "It's starting to shrink."

"It does look better," Tony agreed after a quick peek. He looked thoroughly uncomfortable.

"Let's give it a little longer, and then I'll try to put it back where it belongs."

"Have you had any interesting cases lately?" Jan asked. She sat down on a folding chair Steve placed for her.

I thought for a minute. "Well, I fixed a broken leg on a hamster a while ago. The poor little thing took a tumble down the stairs in his plastic ball." Both Tony and Jan laughed as they pictured the event. "He did really well."

"You mean someone actually paid you to fix a hamster?" Tony asked with an incredulous look on his face. "Why didn't they just step on it and get a new one?"

"I'm going to ignore that comment," I replied. Why do some guys feel the need to be so stupid, I thought. "And I removed a nasalpharyngeal polyp from a cat. That's not something I see every day."

"And again I would ask, why bother?" This time Tony winked as he spoke. Deep wrinkles appeared around his eyes when he smiled. Jan punched his elbow and scowled.

"The rest of the cases have been pretty routine... lumpectomies, spays, neuters and vaccinations." I looked down at the pup. "That is, until tonight when the Reeves arrived."

"Yeah, I'm going to have a hard time explaining this to the guys at the bar," Tony admitted. His face flushed pink again. "This is so embarrassing."

I slipped on a pair of disposable gloves and checked the prepuce. My entire pinky finger now fit between the penis and prepuce. I flushed the sugar solution off of the pup's penis with copious amounts of warm water. With all the dextrose solution gone, I lubed the shaft with KY jelly to reduce friction. With one hand on the penis, I inched the prepuce up the shaft. I pulled on one side and then the other until the penis disappeared back into its protective sleeve.

"He should feel a lot better now," I told his owners. I pushed his penis out again for one last check. A deep red crease encircled the base, but the organ slid back into the prepuce with ease. I removed my gloves and turned off the vaporizer.

Now that everything was in place, I wanted to keep it that way. I told Jan and Tony to separate him from the dominant puppies for a few days until they lost the urge to nurse. Jan agreed to put him in a run with another small pup for company.

"Make sure his penis retracts back into place after he urinates," I continued. "You might need to lube him up and help him along for the first day or so." Jan and Tony looked at each other and laughed. They laughed so hard that tears welled up in their eyes.

"I call that you have to do that," Tony quipped to Jan.

"No way, you're the guy. You have more experience with the equipment than I do," she replied. She stood with her hands on her

hips. Although her head only came to his shoulder, she made a for-
midable image in her faded jeans and boots.

"I wouldn't mess with her, Tony," Steve counseled. "I think
that's a no-win situation."

"See, Steve agrees with me." Jan walked over to Tony and
placed her hand on his shoulder. She kissed him lightly on the
cheek.

"Yes, dear," he responded.

Within two minutes of turning off the vaporizer, the pup began
to twitch. He moved his legs and yipped a few times. I removed
the nose cone. He continued to recover as he breathed in the room
air. A minute later, he lifted his head and gazed at me through
dilated pupils. As I wrapped a towel around him, I bent down and
put my face next to his. The little guy sniffed me and then licked
my cheek. This is the moment I live for as a veterinarian, the feeling
of satisfaction that comes from aiding an animal in need. It makes
the sleepless nights worthwhile.

"Can we go now?" Tony asked, oblivious to the moment I
shared with his puppy.

"Yes," I replied, straightening up. "Just remember to separate
him from the dominant pups and watch him closely." Tony nodded,
picked up the puppy and carried him off like a sack of potatoes.
Although it looked a little rough, the pup didn't seem to mind. He
snuggled into Tony's side.

"Thanks, Kris." Jan looked at Tony. "I knew something was
wrong," she added for effect.

"Yes, dear, you were right, dear," he said as if he had delivered
that line many times. She smiled and placed her arm around his
waist. The two left the clinic arm in arm. I wondered if they would
tell anyone about the events of this night.

CHAPTER 29

Goodbye, Chewy

"Steve, are you ready for a busy day?" I asked as I opened the front door. With the clinic's first anniversary fast approaching, business was good. Patient records filled the shelves behind the reception counter. The slots on the appointment book contained names for several weeks to come. Although the appointment calendar still had blank spaces, it was a great improvement from where we started. The balance in the company checkbook inched upwards. Maybe soon I could start taking a salary.

I rubbed the face of my watch against my shirt. Scratches covered the surface from too many close encounters with the animals. It read 7:30. Saturdays are unpredictable in veterinary medicine. Some are quiet while others are crazy. With most of the appointments slots taken, this looked like a busy one. We hustled to treat all the hospitalized kids before the appointments started.

At 7:45 a.m., the doorbell rang. Steve held a shit tzu on the treatment table. Buster leaned into his body and hid his face under Steve's arm as I inspected the surgical incision on his rear end. Buster's parents divorced earlier in the year. Linda Cooper wanted to stop by early to see Buster before her ex-husband picked him up. It was his week to have the dog.

Steve returned Buster to the first run in the kennel. The shaggy dog spun in circles and knocked over his water bowl. The water ran down the gray concrete floor to the drain. Buster pranced in the water, soaking the fur on his paws.

"Buster," Steve said in disgust. "You stinker! I'll dry off your feet after I see who's up front."

In the lobby, a small blond woman waited at the counter. Curly hair framed her round face and blue eyes. A young girl played in the waiting room, crashing cars together before rolling them off the table onto the floor. When she ran out of cars, she focused her attention on the Disney stickers on the wall. Her little fingers peeled them off with ease. She turned Pongo upside down and placed Perdita on the front window. She grouped the rest of the Dalmatian puppies below their mother on the window.

"Good morning," Steve said as he entered the reception area. "How may I help you?"

"I'm picking up some heartworm preventative for Rusty Baylor," Melanie replied.

"Well it's nice to meet you." He stuck out his right hand. "I'm Steve, Kris husband. She's told me a lot about your family."

"I bet she has." Melanie shook hands with Steve. Just then a loud crash resounded from the play area. "Rachel, I told you to play nice," she scolded.

"It wasn't my fault," the girl replied. "Pongo made the table tip over."

Steve rifled through the items on the shelf behind the counter. Medications in plastic bags filled the space. One by one, Steve looked at the prescription labels until he found a package marked Rusty Baylor. Another crash came from the play area.

"Rachel Catherine Baylor, I told you to play nice." Melanie marched into the kids' area and grabbed the child's arm. She pulled her into the lobby and placed her in a chair by the window. The minute she turned her back, Rachel ran back into the kids' room.

"Uh, Melanie," Steve pointed at the empty chair. Melanie grabbed her again and seated her in the same chair. This time she pointed her finger at the child as she commanded her to stay. Rachel folded her arms across her chest and scowled at her mother. Melanie stared for 10 seconds, then returned to the counter to pay for the medicine. Rachel turned her attention to the Norfolk pine next to her. She ran the soft branches through her fingers. When Melanie wasn't looking, she snapped off the branch.

"Rachel," Steve said in an authoritative voice. "Leave the plant alone."

Melanie turned around to look at her daughter. "That's it. We are not going to the toy store." Rachel's face turned red. She took a deep breath, then screamed. Loud wails filled the clinic. Melanie zipped the medicine into her purse, took Rachel's hand in hers and marched the girl outside. Steve waved through the window, relieved that all of our children were animals.

At precisely 9 a.m., a white van pulled up and parked in front of the clinic. Frank jumped out of the driver's seat clad in his navy blue Customs uniform. Trudy rode in a crate in back. Once Frank gave her the OK command, she leaped out of the vehicle, her tail wagging back and forth in big loops that shook her entire rear end. She loved coming to the vet!

Frank led Trudy directly to the scale. The digital monitor flashed 49.2 pounds. "She is back to her normal weight," Frank announced to Steve. "Now if her blood clots, we are all set." At the six-week check, Trudy's blood test had surprised us all – her clotting time was still prolonged. I had placed her on another three weeks of vitamin K1. We all hoped it would be her last dose.

As the test ran, Frank demonstrated Trudy's ability to find drugs. He hid two training boxes in the clinic, one in a pharmacy cabinet and the other in between bags of prescription dog food. He brought Trudy back into the room and gave the search command. Trudy sprang into action. She started at one end of the room with Frank trailing behind her. Two feet past the cabinet containing the box, she stopped dead in her tacks. Her nose swung back toward the cabinet. She sniffed the front, scratched the door and sat down in front of it.

"Good girl, Trudy." Frank pulled the rolled-up towel from his back pocket. Trudy jumped up and grabbed it with her teeth. The two played tug-of-war for a minute. "Good girl, Trudy. You're a good girl," he continued to praise her. Eventually, Frank released his grip on the towel, and Trudy trotted around the room, displaying her prize proudly. She looked great. Frank called her back and clipped the lead onto her collar. Again, he gave the search command. Trudy continued where she left off. When she reached the food storage area, she zeroed in on the lower shelf. Two sniffs later, she found the second box.

The timer dinged a minute after Trudy finished her demonstration. I crossed my fingers on my left hand as I slowly inverted the tube. The blood stayed firmly in place at the top, forming a hard clot that would not budge.

"Congratulations, Frank," I said holding the tube in my hand. "She's back to normal." Frank knelt down and hugged Trudy. She rested her head on his shoulder and licked his neck. She was not sure why he was hugging her, but she certainly loved it.

"Before I go, I need to ask you one last favor, Dr. Nelson." The seriousness of Frank's voice made me freeze. "Would you mind writing a report about this?"

"A report?" I asked. "What kind of report?"

At the same time Trudy got sick, two other Customs dogs on the border suddenly stopped working. They eventually died. The FBI launched a formal investigation into the matter to determine if the two events were related or simply a coincidence. Frank hoped the results would clear him of any wrongdoing. He pulled an official envelope out of his pocket. They wanted a copy of Trudy's medical record as well as my opinion on the matter.

"Frank, you weren't negligent." I patted his arm. He continued to look at the ground. "In my experience, dogs that get into a small amount of rat bait, even the long-acting stuff, don't need nine weeks of therapy. I don't think she grabbed a mouthful when you were searching a warehouse. I think she ate a large amount, which means someone poisoned her on purpose." Frank looked up at me with an intense look. "I've been suspicious since the three-week check. The death of the dogs on the border confirms my feelings. I'm just glad they used something I could treat."

"Really." Frank stared into my eyes.

"Yes, she's the first patient I've ever had that didn't clot at all at the three-week recheck." I looked at Trudy. "And the first patient I've had to treat for nine weeks. I think she ate a ton of poison. This wasn't an accident." Frank stood up straight. A gleam returned to his eyes.

"Thanks, Dr. Nelson." He shook my hand. "I appreciate your help."

Ten minutes after Frank and Trudy left, a bright red pickup truck with dual back wheels pulled into the parking lot. The chrome spokes sparkled as the truck rolled to a stop. More chrome framed the license plates, which declared "Minnesota Land of Ten Thousand Lakes." Dad hopped out of the driver's seat in a short-sleeve shirt with a thermos of coffee in one hand and his tool belt in the other.

"Hi, Dad," I greeted him as he walked into the treatment room. I knelt in front of the treatment table with a syringe in my hand. Steve held a fluffy white cat on the table with his front legs over the edge. The cat swished his tail back and forth.

"What are you two doing?" Dad asked.

"I need some blood from this cat. Unfortunately, Fluffy is not cooperating." I sprayed more rubbing alcohol on his neck and smoothed down the hair. "Steve, on the count of three, blow into his face." I removed the cap from the needle. "One." I pressed my fingers into his neck. His left jugular swelled. "Two." I held the syringe up to his neck. Steve inhaled deeply. "Three." I poked the syringe through the skin as Steve blew. Fluffy growled but did not move. Blood rushed into the syringe from the large vein.

Fluffy's growls turned into death threats. "I'm not sure I can hold him like this much longer," Steve announced between puffs. "Hurry!"

"Just a little more," I replied. Fluffy screamed. Saliva dripped from his lips onto my hand. Fluffy managed to free one of his front legs from Steve's grasp.

"Watch out," Steve yelled. Fluffy extended his claws and swiped at my hand. I pulled away just in time to feel the air rush by my skin. "Whew, that was a close one." Steve regained control of the cat and applied pressure to the venipuncture site. Two minutes later, he placed Fluffy's carrier on the table. Fluffy looked around for a second, then bolted inside. From the safety of his carrier, we heard a deep rumble.

"Oh, enough already." Steve closed the door and carried the angry cat back to his owner.

"You have a full waiting room up front, Kris," Dad commented. "Business must be good."

"Yeah, we've been busy." I smiled at my Dad. "It's changed a lot since that first day. Remember when you and I walked into this place? It was a disaster."

"Don't remind me," he replied. "Your business made a lot of work for me." He looked around the treatment room. The cabinet door under the scrub sink was open, and a bright yellow bucket sat beneath the pipes. He removed his tool belt and lay down on his back with his head inside the cabinet. I returned to the pharmacy for my next appointment.

Since her last visit, Chewy, the gerbil, had lived like a princess, enjoying the special treatment her young owner lavished on her. Billy spent every minute he could with his little friend. The gerbil enjoyed extra time in her plastic ball, exploring her environment. When she finished, Billy rewarded her with her favorite treats. Afterwards, she curled up for a nap in the pocket of his hoodie. Life was great until yesterday – when she stopped eating.

Inside the cat room, Billy sat on the chair with Chewy in his arms. His eyes were red and swollen. Jill stood by his side with her hand on her son's shoulder. She instructed him to put Chewy on the table for her examination.

"Oh, that's OK. I'll examine her in your arms." I exchanged places with Jill and knelt beside the boy. Chewy looked horrible. A dull scruffy coat replaced her sleek brown fur. Her eyes looked dull, too. She had lost a tremendous amount of weight; I could not feel any subcutaneous fat anywhere. When I ran my finger down the leg with the tumor, it felt like all her muscle was gone. The tumor had doubled in size since her last visit. She held her leg off the ground and was careful not to lie on it.

I watched her for a minute before placing my stethoscope on her chest. Her sides heaved in and out in rapid succession. Through the eartips I heard abnormal crackles and pops. Her inquisitive personality evaporated as she struggled for air. I placed the bell against the other side of her chest, and my heart sank.

"I'm hearing some abnormal sounds in her chest." I replaced the stethoscope around my neck. I stroked Chewy's head and stood up. A heavy silence filled the room.

"Do you think the tumor has spread?" Jill asked.

I swallowed hard before answering. "That's what I'm afraid of." I looked down at the gerbil cuddled into Billy's arms. "But we need to take an X-ray to make sure it's not something I can treat, like pneumonia."

"Go ahead and take the X-ray," Jill said. "Billy and I will wait outside in the car."

I reached my hands toward Chewy. Billy hugged her as tears rolled down his cheeks. "Give Chewy to Dr. Nelson," Jill instructed her son. Billy kissed the gerbil on the forehead, held her another 30 seconds and then placed her in my hands.

Fifteen minutes later, the X-rays confirmed my worst fears. Cancer filled Chewy's lungs. I couldn't find any normal areas. I held Chewy against my chest as Steve went to get her family. She felt so frail. The cancer seemed to devour her body right in front of my eyes.

Jill looked at me and knew immediately that the news was not good. She placed her arm around her son's shoulders and held a tissue to her nose. Billy looked at me with eager eyes. He hoped beyond hope that I would be able to help his friend. I took a deep breath. This was the part of my job that I dread.

"I'm afraid it's not good," I told him as I handed Chewy to him. Instead of sniffing his face like normal, she just lay in his arms. I pointed to her lungs on the X-ray. "The tumor on her leg has metastasized to her lungs. See all the white lumps?" Jill stared at the film in silence.

"Is she suffering?" Jill whispered.

"Yes, she can't breathe because the tumor has destroyed most of her lung tissue."

Jill knelt down in front of her son and drew him near. Billy buried his face on her shoulder and wept. I dabbed at my eyes with a tissue. Dad stopped his work under the sink. He looked at me and pulled a handkerchief out of his pocket.

"We do not want her to suffer," Jill said, still hugging her son. "We love her too much for that."

I nodded in response. "I'll anesthetize Chewy, and then I'll give her a drug that stops her heart. She won't feel a thing. She'll just fall asleep." I tried to smile reassuringly. "Then after she's gone, you can take her body home with you, or I can cremate her for you."

"We talked about it in the car." Jill looked at her son. "We would like to keep Chewy's ashes with us so we never forget her." The boy nodded, his face wet with tears.

"You'll never forget Chewy. She will always hold a special place in your heart," I replied.

Jill cleared her throat. "Billy, it's time to give Chewy to Dr. Nelson." Billy stared into his mother's eyes for a few seconds. He drew the gerbil close to his heart and kissed her on the head. She reached up and touched his face with her nose, like she did when she was healthy. Then she collapsed in his arms.

"Please take good care of her, Dr. Nelson," Billy whispered. "Tell her that I love her and that she's the best gerbil in the world." I nodded and blinked back the tears. Billy placed her in my hands and kissed her again. "Bye, Chewy, I love you."

Jill wiped tears from her eyes. She kissed her finger and touched Chewy's head with it. "Thank you for taking such good care of Chewy," she said to me. The words pierced my heart like a knife. I could never understand why clients thanked me for ending their pet's life. To me, euthanasia always felt like defeat. I forced a smile in response.

Jill hugged her son and escorted him out of the room. As soon as they left the building, I hooked up the anesthesia machine. I placed Chewy inside the large dog nose cone. She lay on her side without exploring the unfamiliar environment. Within a minute of turning on the gas, she slept. As the gas continued to flow, Chewy's respirations slowed until her chest stopped moving. I removed her limp body from the cone.

"Rest in peace, little Chewy. Your family loves you very much." Dad joined me at the treatment table as I gave the final injection. "You are the best gerbil in the world." I wrapped her up in a towel and placed her inside a plastic bag. In big black letters I wrote, "Chewy Carlson, Private Cremation" across the front.

I looked at my Dad. "And that is the worst part of being a veterinarian," I said. Dad nodded. He patted the plastic bag, then returned to the sink without saying a word.

Dealing with death is a big part of veterinary medicine. Veterinarians must find a way to process death, or their careers will be short-lived. For me, the best medicine is to spend time with another animal. I walked into my office and found Genny asleep on the office chair. I closed the door and knelt beside her. In the privacy of the office, I buried my face in her fur and cried. I cried for Chewy and all the other animals I euthanized over my career.

Genny looked at me with sleepy eyes. Although she didn't understand why, she knew I was upset and wanted to help. She placed one of her front paws on my cheek. A second later, she started to purr. It was exactly what I needed.

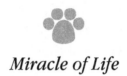

CHAPTER 30

Miracle of Life

After losing Chewy, fate blessed me with the perfect gift to lift my spirit – the creation of life with two adorable golden retrievers. Goldens are among the happiest dogs on earth. They rarely seem to have a bad day and live with gusto. Give them a ball, and they play for hours. Give them the same dry dog food day after day, and they wolf it down in less than a minute. Give them love, and they return it tenfold.

When I emerged from the office, a large golden named Sam waited for me in the pharmacy/laboratory area. He sat patiently by his owner, Ron Evans, who leaned against the counter dressed in khaki shorts and a golf shirt. On the counter next to him was a package of sterile gloves, a long pipette and a heating pad. An artificial vagina and test tube warmed beneath the pad.

"Good morning, Ron," I greeted him, trying to hide the emotion of losing Chewy moments before. Sam stood at attention with a gleam in his eye. His tail thumped against the cabinets. "And good morning to you, handsome." Sam's deep rust-colored fur reminded me of a dog I grew up with. "Are you ready for fun?" The dog watched me intensely – he knew what was coming.

"Is the bitch here yet?" Ron asked without returning my greeting. "Mitch promised he would drop her off early this morning." I nodded. "Then what are we waiting for? Let's get this over with." He looked at the stunning gold watch on his wrist. "I have a tee time at noon." I nodded again. Ron was always in a hurry. In the summer it was golf, in the winter it was racquetball. This man was always late for something.

I grabbed a leash from the treatment room and headed to the kennel. Ashley waited for her date with Sam.

"Come here, Ashley," I called, and she bounded into my arms. Instead of the more common dark gold color, Ashley's hair was fair. Her black nose and dark brown eyes stood out against her blond fur. I placed the leash around her neck and led her out of the kennel.

Dad stood next to the counter with a wrench in one hand and a pipe in the other. Cleaning supplies from under the sink sat next to him. More tools littered the floor. For this procedure, I needed his help. After one look at the blond bombshell, he eagerly left his tools behind. Fortunately, Dad did not ask why I wanted his help.

"This is my Dad, Ron," I said introducing them to each other. "He's going to help so we can get you on your way." I handed Ashley's leash to Steve. Ron nodded at my dad and looked at his watch again. Steve walked Ashley to the middle of the room so Sam would have plenty of space. It wasn't a honeymoon suite in Vegas, but it gave him room to maneuver and provided all the ambience Sam needed.

Steve kneeled on the floor next to Ashley with his hands on her collar. I removed the artificial vagina from the heating pad and attached the warm test tube.

"Ready?" Ron asked. I nodded. He walked Sam over to Ashley and pointed at her swollen vulva. Sam sniffed. She immediately flagged, her tail raised high in the air and held off to the side. Sam wagged his tail and yipped. He understood her communication. She wanted him, and he was delighted to oblige. Sam licked her vulva. She flagged even more. Love at first sight.

I knelt down beside Ashley's rear end with the collection apparatus in my hands. Sam looked at me and mounted her back. With my dad watching and clearly uncomfortable at the sight of his daughter on her knees participating in this event, I quickly positioned the artificial vagina over Sam's penis. Sam thrust his body forward. Four quick pushes later, milky liquid filled the test tube. He dismounted Ashley with a grin that was beyond silly. I peeled the artificial vagina off his engorged penis.

"Wow, that's a big sample," I exclaimed, much to Ron's delight.

"Yeah, he's always been a good breeder," Ron said with a huge smile on his face. He gathered the leash in his hand. "Are we done?"

"Almost – let me take a quick peek at the semen under the microscope." I walked over to the counter where my dad stood. "Dad, hold this." I detached the test tube from the artificial vagina. "You need to keep the sample warm while I check it." Dad's usually steady hand trembled as he reached for the test tube, his face bright red. I placed a drop of semen on a warm slide, positioned it under the microscope and began the analysis. Silence filled the room as three men awaited my verdict.

The entire slide vibrated with sperm. Their tails whipped back and forth as they struggled toward an unseen goal. Most swam in straight lines across the field of view. My eyes scanned for problems such as heads detached from tails or swimming in circles. I found no issues. The sperm were sound and sturdy. Out of hundreds on the slide, I detected only two bent tails, a minor problem.

"Looks good," I announced and turned off the microscope. "He's got great motility with only a few secondary defects." Ron stood even taller. He absolutely glowed. He stroked Sam's head, as proud of his stud as if this breeding reflected his own talent.

"Can I go now?" he asked.

"I'd rather you wait until his erection subsides. He's still hanging kind of low." I previously had one unfortunate injury when a dog hurt himself jumping into a truck.

Ron looked at Sam's swollen penis. The golden walked with his back legs wide apart to accommodate the size. Long after his thrusts into the artificial vagina in my hands, clear prostatic fluid still dripped onto the floor of the clinic.

"Not to worry, Dr. Nelson," he insisted. "I'll take good care of him. See you later."

With the collection and analysis complete, I turned my attention to Ashley. I put on sterile gloves before touching the pipette and syringe, then motioned to my dad. He walked over to me with the test tube clutched tightly in his right hand. Unable to look at me, he kept his eyes fixed on the floor. I inserted the pipette into the test tube and aspirated Sam's semen. When every drop of the precious material was in the syringe, I instructed Dad to hold Ashley's tail out of the way. He did as I asked, all without any eye contact. I giggled inside.

I gently inserted a gloved finger and the tip of the pipette through the lips of the vulva. Ashley's rear end sank to the ground. Evidently, I was no substitute for Sam.

"No, no," Steve sprang to action. "You have to stand for this, sweetie." He pulled her up to her feet. She tried to sit again but could not with Steve's hand under her abdomen. I reinserted the pipette and slid it down her vagina into place. A quick push on the syringe plunger sent the sperm hurtling toward the eggs. Perhaps the miracle of life would soon begin. I detached the syringe, filled it with air and flushed the pipette twice before removing it from her body.

Now began the wait. To help the sperm find their target, the female's hips need to be elevated for 20 minutes. Steve knew the drill from assisting me with other inseminations. He placed a white rubber stepstool under her rear legs to let gravity go to work. The stool elevated Ashley's hips above her head. She swung her head around for a better look at the stool. She could understand neither why the sex was so unfulfilling, nor why we humans were making her stand in such an awkward position.

I gave Steve and my dad folding chairs to make the wait more comfortable. They set the chairs on either side of Ashley, Steve holding her collar while Dad held onto her back. A stifling silence ensued. Dad continued to stare at the floor, and Steve looked at the clock on the wall. Neither said a word. Ashley had 18 minutes to go.

My father is a traditional guy. He worked hard to provide for our family while my mother stayed home to care for us kids. Sunday morning, they loaded us into the family sedan for church. Dad always drove while my mother primped in the mirror on the passenger visor. They followed the teachings of the church – no alcohol, tobacco, swearing or gambling. They also frowned on dancing and any movie without a G rating. The topic of sex was strictly off-limits. I had a safe, comfortable and strict upbringing.

I was totally clueless about sex. I knew it took a male and a female, but that was the extent of my knowledge for many years. We moved from Hopkins to a farm when I was 12, and that was my first true exposure to breeding. After wrapping the mare's tail, the adults always made me leave the barn before the stallion arrived. I peeked through the door, but never saw the good stuff. About the only thing I learned is that breeding horses is noisy, and stallions seem to like it.

One year, I decided we should have baby rabbits, but my mother disagreed. She believed the two we had were sufficient. After school, I snuck down to the barn and put the doe into the buck's cage. As I watched, the doe flattened her body against the cage floor. She lay motionless except for wrinkling her nose. The buck uttered low-pitched guttural sounds as he jumped to and fro over her back. I recall wondering how in the world this led to babies.

After a few minutes of bored observation, I returned the doe to her cage, and a month later, she gave birth to a large litter of bunnies. Mom did not accept my explanation of divine intervention. Perhaps she knew more about this process than I thought. I learned two important lessons from this experience. First, never underestimate the reproductive capabilities of rabbits. Second, never under-estimate the wrath of a mother disobeyed.

Today, the silence between the men holding Ashley remained deafening. Finally, Steve felt obligated to lower the tension, choosing a light approach. "Well, Gordy, did you ever think you would see your daughter do that?"

Dad chuckled nervously and shook his head. He looked at Steve for the first time since the breeding began. "I never thought she'd ask me to hold the sample, either." With that, my Dad and my husband erupted in laughter. They laughed so long and so hard their faces turned red.

"I have to admit," Steve said, pausing to catch his breath, "When we got married, I didn't plan on ever doing this with my father-in-law."

"And I never thought I'd be doing this with my son-in-law," my dad replied. "Let's not tell Kris' mother." They laughed some more. I enjoyed seeing them together. Good but very different men by profession and nature, they found common ground through the breeding of two golden retrievers. The cloud of sadness that hung over the clinic with the death of Chewy lifted.

The tension broken, the two most important men in my life discussed safe topics; the weather, the Minnesota Twins and family. Eventually the conversation turned to business. With the first anniversary of the clinic just days away, Dad wanted to know how things were going. Although he never said it out loud, he wondered if I could really run a business. In his mind, I was still his little girl.

Steve excitedly described the growth of the practice. He recounted being concerned in the early months when we hoped for just one precious appointment per day. Now we looked back fondly on the spring heartworm season when the clinic finally broke-even. We feared business would slow down over the summer, but revenue remained strong. Now, at our first anniversary, we could hire more help. "We're going to add another technician as soon as Kris finds the right one," Steve told my Dad.

Steve looked at the clock and counted off the last 60 seconds. "Good girl," Steve praised Ashley. He released his grip on her collar. Dad let go, too. She stepped off the stool and pranced around.

My dad stood up and hugged me. A Navy man and contractor by trade, he was not prone to emotion. But today, Dad said he was proud of me and the practice. I felt tears welling again, but this time, tears of joy. My dream came true. Wouldn't Dr. Anderson be thrilled.

Acknowledgments

Wh_

When my friend heard I was writing a book, she told me that "writing a book is like living in the desert and the oasis keeps moving." Since I live in the desert, her words resonated with my soul and the experience of writing. Thank goodness, as I wrote, I have been surrounded by animals.

Let me start by thanking a gifted editor, Deb Rinard, for making the words disappear as the stories came to life. She did more than correct mistakes. Deb made the book more readable while keeping my voice intact. Her editorial expertise, combined with tangible love for her own cats, Snicker and Doodle, made her the perfect editor for this book. In addition, she has been a joy to work with.

My sincere thanks to Vickie Mullins and Brandi Hollister of Mullins Creative for illuminating my ideas in these pages. The firm's professionalism and skill in book design are a great gift to an author. Miniature pinchers Tinkerbell and Jasmine no doubt contributed to the flair and focus Mullins Creative brought to this project.

To my literary attorney, Jonathan Kirsch, a heartfelt thanks for all of his advice. Jonathan has guided me over several years as I set up my company, developed a media presence and finally, wrote a book. Thanks for your wise counsel and encouragement, Jonathan.

When it came time to shoot a picture for the back cover, I called photographer Tina Celle. In addition to years of experience, Tina lives with Foxy, a lovely Pomeranian. She patiently positioned my pets – Mauka the cat, and Buddy the dog – and encouraged them to look at the camera. Thankfully, Tina has patience without measure.

Dara Rybalov is a gifted artist and designed the book's cover. At first sight, I loved her work! Dara is passionate about art and books so this was a perfect marriage of her talent and interest. Thank you, Dara. Her creative process is enhanced by two Siamese cats, Ming and LeMei, who insist she take regular breaks from designing to play fetch.

Throughout the last year family and friends have been asking about the book. "How's it going? When will it be published?" I wondered the same thing myself on several occasions.... . Thanks for your constant support, words of encouragement and inspiration. I hope the finished work was worth the wait!

Writing is an exercise in solitude. Yet I never felt alone or that this was a solo endeavor. Thank you to my husband, Steve, for his untiring enthusiasm and belief in me. Thanks, too, for all your help with the clinic and now with the book. I'm glad I worked so hard to get that first date 23 years ago!

Last, my heartfelt thanks to all the clients who trusted me with their beloved pets. I know animals are cherished members of your family. It is a privilege and honor to care for them. Their stories live forever in my heart!

About the Author

D r. Kristen Nelson grew up on a farm in Watertown, Minnesota, where she developed a deep love for animals of all kinds. She received a Doctor of Veterinary Medicine degree from the University of Minnesota, College of Veterinary Medicine. Kris then completed a small-animal internship at the prestigious Animal Medical Center in New York City.

In addition to writing and speaking, she cares for small and exotic animals in Scottsdale, Arizona. Dr. Nelson is widely quoted in the media. Her credits include *USA TODAY, The Los Angeles Times,* DisneyFamily.com and numerous radio and television interviews. Kris and her husband, Steve, share their home with rescued cats, birds and a dog.

More information about Dr. Nelson is available at www.veterinarycreative.com. Dr. Nelson answers veterinary questions at www.drnelsonsveterinaryblog.com. You may also follow her on Facebook and Twitter. For those seeking admission to professional college, she offers advice and has guides available for purchase at: www.vetschoolapp.com,   www.medschoolapp.com,   and www.dentschoolapp.com.

CPSIA information can be obtained at www.ICGtesting.com
Printed in the USA
BVOW08s2124190516

448562BV00001B/28/P